ABC

ABC's of Natural Healing:

Better Health for You and the Planet

through

Amazon Rainforest Herbs

By

Terra Mar

Terra Mar

Copyright © 2009 by Terra Mar.

All rights reserved. Reproduction and distribution are forbidden. No part of this publication may be reproduced, stored in a retrieval system, or transmitted by any other means, electronic, mechanical, photocopying, recording, or otherwise, without written permission from the author. Please contact terra@oneplanetherbs.com.

The author and publisher have used their best efforts in preparing this book and shall in no event be held liable for any loss or damages including but not limited to special, incidental, or consequential.

ISBN 978-0-578-01428-9

Published by Macro Connections Publishing, a division of Macro Connections, LLC.

Cover design by Katherin Scott

On beginning this journey of ABC simplicity

Remarks by His Holiness the Dalai Lama, from his Nobel speech in Oslo, 1989

"Because we all share this small planet Earth, we have to learn to live in harmony and peace with each other and with nature. That is not just a dream, but a necessity...

The realization that we are all basically the same human beings, who seek happiness and try to avoid suffering, is very helpful in developing a sense of brotherhood and sisterhood – a warm feeling of love and compassion for others.

This, in turn, is essential if we are to survive in this ever shrinking world we live in. For if we each selfishly pursue only what we believe to be in our own interest, without caring about the needs of others, we not only may end up harming others but also ourselves.

I speak to you as just another human being – as a simple monk. If you find what I say useful, then I hope you will try to practice it."

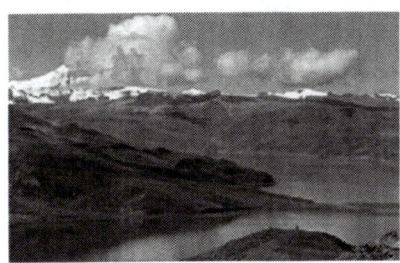

Terra Mar

Introduction to the A B C's of the Amazon Rainforest:

A is for Amazon

B is for breath

C is for caring

Introducing you to the greatest herbs of all time is my passion. But first I have to introduce the master of ceremonies, the Amazon Rainforest.

The Amazon Rainforest is a Big Deal. It really is.

Big in size. It covers parts of 9 countries in South America and is about the size of the lower U.S. 48 states *combined*.

Big in what it has to offer. We're used to thinking a geographical treasure belongs to a place, like the Everglades to Florida or the Grand Canyon to Colorado. That's not the way it is with the Amazon. For one thing, the Amazon is literally a part of you and me. Since it protects 20 percent of the oxygen we breathe you could say with every fifth intake of air, we breathe in one of its gifts.

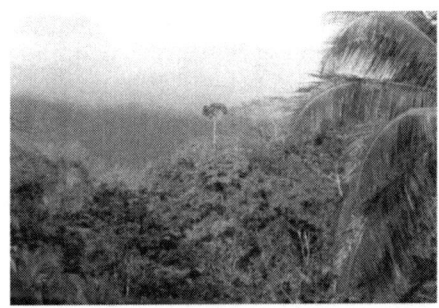

The Amazon is also the container for a fifth of all the fresh water on earth. It's got the greatest biodiversity of anywhere on the planet. One in ten known species of flora and fauna live in the Amazon Rainforest. That's the world's largest living species repository. (World Wildlife Fund)

There's more. Much more. It's the source of most of our wonder drugs for heart and cancer and many of our western pharmaceuticals. The U.S. National Cancer Institute has identified 2000 plants with anti-cancer properties, 70% of these are found only in the rainforest. (The Nature Conservancy). From an herbal standpoint it is Mecca.

Terra Mar

Big in trouble

Deforestation is what happens to a rainforest when some people's shortsighted greed and other people's desperation intersect. The resulting destruction of an irreplaceable resource the world desperately needs is staggering. Some 4,600 sq. 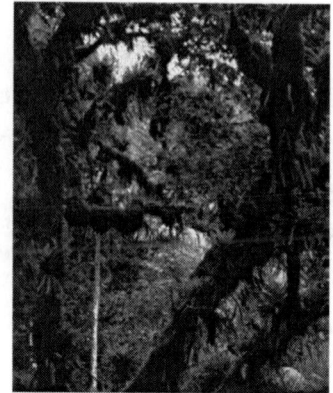 miles of the Amazon rainforest were destroyed in 2008. (Mongabay). That's the equivalent of taking an axe to almost the entire state of Connecticut.

The Nature Conservancy did the math as well. We're currently destroying a football field of rainforest every *second*. Each year that's 31 million football fields of rainforest gone forever. WWF says that unless we stop current practices, 55 percent of the Amazon rainforest will be gone by 2030.

I know you care. But what can you do?

Maybe more than you think. Did you know that if the rainforest is destroyed the human race will not survive?

Here's an exercise. Think of someone you love who needed blood thinner or cancer medication or heart medicine or quinine so they wouldn't get malaria while travelling. I don't want you to think of what would have happened if they hadn't gotten it. That's too nasty. I just want you to savor and appreciate how it helped.

That too is a reminder of why we care. So much of the herbal bounty of the rainforest is yet to be discovered. Only fractions of the species have been named, far fewer studied. So much potential healing.

So, what can you do? You can go online and pick your rainforest preservation group. Donate. Buy a bit of land. Find a social organization that works with indigenous economies and buy from them. Buy rainforest herbs that utilize social projects in the Amazon. Write to your Senator. Travel to the Rainforest and fall in love with it.

Find your own way, and then whatever it is, own it. Protect-an-Acre (https://secure.ga3.org/03/ran_PAA_Gift) is a grants program that contributes directly to rainforest communities struggling to protect the natural-resource base on which they and we rely. At their web site you can pay as little as $1.00 to begin helping.

Maybe the most important way to help is the easiest. Share your knowledge and concerns. Talk to your family, friends and colleagues. Help them to turn caring into action. They want to breathe too.

Terra Mar

Suggestions for using this book

My intent in writing this ABC book is twofold – first to place natural health and healing in the context of Nature itself. If you rethink some of the assumptions about your place in the biosphere or on your block, I'll be happy.

Secondly, I want to introduce you to some of the most influential herbs of all time – healing herbs from the Amazon Rainforest.

You don't have to read in any particular order; feel free to open to whatever jumps out at you. Random is good. Each letter stands alone, although each is part of a Weltanschauung that views us as part of the web Nature has woven for us all.

Each chapter ends with a takeaway -- an exercise, a fun activity, or questions to contemplate and discuss. It is my hope that you and the words will interact with each other, that your imagination will take what you see a step further, and that in some way you'll be moved to action.

I also hope you will keep a journal on some of your activities rather than writing them in various places. Alternately write, scribble or journal all over these pages. It helps make it your own.

Disclaimer

An enormous amount of research has gone into this book. Not only my own, but that of indigenous healers and western scientists. None of it is meant to substitute for your own wisdom, research, self-knowledge and contact with health care professionals. As you read about these wonderful healing herbs, please bear in mind that what you are learning is for information purposes only. Nothing in this book is intended to diagnose, prescribe, or administer in any manner to any ailment. In matters related to your health, please contact a qualified healthcare practitioner.

The herb descriptions are compiled from a variety of sources I deemed reliable, but may contain omissions or errors in fact, or become outdated.

Where references are made to traditional uses this is not intended as any medical claims about the ability or efficacy of any of these plants to treat, prevent, cure or mitigate any disease or condition.

This book is not designed as a scientific work and is not intended in any way to cover, review or analyze the efficacy of scientific research that may exist for any plant mentioned.

Terra Mar

Acknowledgment and dedication

Reading acknowledgements for me is like watching an auto accident. I don't want to look, and I do it anyway. Being on the other side at the moment I feel a grudging respect for anyone who can tease out who to acknowledge and thank for a book.

I'm unable to see where it began. I could try your patience and start with the girls who ignored me in grade school, but I won't.

Instead I'll spare the space and use a broad brush, trying neither to omit nor to bore. First my gratitude goes to all of the people, places, and things seen and unseen, acknowledged and not, that have nudged, prodded, pulled, insisted and dragged me to this moment.

This book is a compendium not only of herbs and information, but of my experiences, passions, victories and losses. I am grateful to all for different reasons.

I am grateful to the teachers and healers – plants and human – that have sustained us since the veiled beginnings of time and will be with us as long as there is life.

I want to acknowledge the amazing body of research developed by Dr. Leslie Taylor, naturopath, fountain of knowledge on rainforest herbs, owner of Raintree Nutrition (www.rain-tree.com) and trusted source from whom I source herbs for my company.

To people I carry in my heart and who carry me through the rough patches:

Hanshi 10th Dan, Isao Ichikawa, a teacher like no other, an indelible spirit that inhabited a body for too short a time, and whose profound connection to Nature inspired me to find my own. If I have incorporated any wisdom, it's likely from you. I owe you more than I can possibly say. Perhaps you would be proud that I write this small acknowledgement, 13 years to the day since you passed on.

My sister, who still laughs and loves with abandon and her beloved Ira, who would have been humbled to be acknowledged -- then made a joke.

My friends, you know who you are and how important you are to me. You too are in these pages, (for better or worse) with love and remembrance. I rely on you all.

The seventh generation. We struggle to imagine you yet we will be your ancestors. I want you to remember us as the generation that said "yes we can" and then did.

Finally, the three most important men in my life. I would never have known the magic but for you.

This mosaic is for, and in great part from, all of you.

Terra Mar

Table of Contents

On beginning this journey of ABC simplicity — i

Introduction to the A B C's of the Rainforest — ii

Suggestions for using this book — vi

Disclaimer — vii

Acknowledgment and Dedication — viii

A is for Aphrodisiac — 1

B is for Bitters — 8

C is for Curanderos — 14

D is for Disease — 19

E is for Ethnobotany — 24

F is for Fatigue — 31

G is for Gaia — 37

H is for Herbs — 45

I is for Immune — 52

J is for Jatobá — 59

K is for Kidneys — 63

L is for Lungs — 68

M is for Menopause — 74

N is for Nature — 81

O is for Obesity — 88

P is for Pacing — 96

Q is for Quechua — 104

R is for Remedies — 112

S is for Sleep — 120

T is for Trees — 129

U is for Upset — 137

V is for Virus — 145

W is for Wounds — 153

X is for ? (the X factor) — 160

Y is for Yeast — 164

Z is for Zen — 172

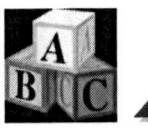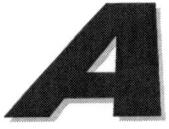 is for Aphrodisiac

"The moon is nothing but a circumambulating aphrodisiac divinely subsidized to provoke the world into a rising birth-rate." -- **Christopher Fry**, English Writer (1907-2005)

You've heard the term, maybe tried some yourself. So what is an aphrodisiac?

The derivation is from Aphrodite, the Greek goddess of sensuality and love. I already like it. An aphrodisiac is commonly defined as any substance that heightens sexual interest and sexual desire. My definition is similar with a twist: For me an aphrodisiac is a substance that helps get our body into a sexy state of harmony and balance.

Throughout history certain plants, drinks and foods have been considered natural aphrodisiacs. Some have been quick fads; others have long histories of use. Many have stayed with us for millennia and remain an irrepressible testimonial to our fascination with enhancing the sexual experience.

Foods that have long been considered aphrodisiacs include asparagus, bananas, chocolate, figs, honey, and oysters, to name a few. Still others are aphrodisiacs because of their intoxicating aromas. Think almond,

Terra Mar

anise, jasmine, nutmeg or vanilla. Some have attained this lofty status from reputation. Others fall into the 'Doctrine of Signatures.' That means what the plant 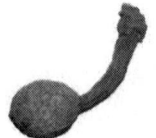 part looks like in relation to the human body is the part it will help. A classic example is ginseng root, which looks like a person and is a proven tonic. Now if you look at this picture of huanarpo macho that should tell you something... Smile.

Why go *herbal* for aphrodisiacs?

In a word or two -- good health. For serious aphrodisiac hunters this is where the rubber meets the road, so to speak. With the advent of Viagra, Levitra and Cialis, men's desire to overcome erectile dysfunction, enhance potency, and increase libido became a marketing hit. You may already know that Viagra was originally created to lower blood pressure. Then some keen observers noticed this other thing happening as well, and a new industry burst on the scene.

All was well until many of the serious side effects of these pharmaceuticals became known. That helped open the marketing for herbal solutions.

Herbs are not only aphrodisiacs with a longer history of use, but are vastly more complex aphrodisiacs. I mean that in a good way. In contrast to a synthesized component in a pharmaceutical, the herbs are a complete gift. They pass along their complex balance that has helped them survive and thrive as a living being in harmony with nature. Sexual vitality, pleasure and functionality for both men and women are also complex. This is bringing like to like, a complex solution to a complex situation.

At the physiological level there is a lot going on when it comes to sexual feelings and performance. This includes a strong libido based in good energy levels, balanced hormones, a strong flow of blood to the genitals, a balanced nervous system, and physiological relaxation.

Looked at that way you could wonder how any of us 21st centuryites could possibly have healthy libidos. But we do, and generally those of us interested in aphrodisiacs already have good sex. We just want more frequency, even better sex, or a specially enhanced experience.

The best kept secret of herbal aphrodisiacs

Switching gears into anything worthwhile from a high stress job, taking care of kids, or being glued to a computer screen all day isn't easy. Transforming into a potent superman or femme fatale may work in the movies, or the early stages of a romance, but it's hard on a day-to-day basis. Despite that, for the really good stuff to get rolling we need to be in the mood.

What aphrodisiacs do is help us make that switch by helping us *relax*. That's actually the secret ingredient in herbal aphrodisiacs. It's the nervous system's equivalent of dimming the lights, putting on soft music and clicking the champagne glasses together.

If you look at the list of top herbal aphrodisiacs they all share in common the ability to make us feel gooood. They soothe and relax the central nervous system. They get the blood flowing. They increase hormone levels of the happy stuff -- like serotonin and dopamine. They relax our muscles, and increase our health by helping our body into a sexy state of harmony and balance.

Incomplete science; lots of history

With many herbs scientific research is either incomplete or has barely begun. That's a long story and different topic about how and why we research plants. More to our topic: what some of these aphrodisiac herbs lack in scientific validation, they make up for in anecdotal use over many centuries and continued preference in modern herbal formulae.

Maybe there will come a time when science finds a way to increase funding for public interest research into healing plants. Unfortunately we're not there yet and pharmaceutical companies often seek to validate only parts of plants they can patent.

Meanwhile, please remember that the following descriptions, like all others in this book are for information purposes only.

These are considered some of the best herbal aphrodisiacs from the Amazon rainforest:

Catuaba (*Erythroxylum catuaba*) has been used for hundreds of years in the rainforest, and is now found in aphrodisiacs in the U.S. Although it has a long and proven track record as an aphrodisiac and for other uses, no negative side effects have been reported. Some come and go; this one's a keeper. Catuaba also has a reputation for inducing erotic dreams. LOL's.

Damiana (*Tumera aphrodisiaca*) The Mayans and Aztecs used damiana as an aphrodisiac, and its use continues today. "Aphrodisiac" is literally in the species name - *Tumera aphrodisiaca*. Some scientific evidence has also weighed in on damiana. It is often recommended for improved sleep. More laughs about sweet dreams.

Huanarpo macho (*Jatropha macrantha*) is probably the best known of Peru's natural aphrodisiacs for men. It is widely believed that it can help prevent premature ejaculation and erectile dysfunction, and can function as an overall male sexual tonic. Though not scientifically proven, I can see where the name might appeal to guys.

Maca (*Lepidium meyenii*) is a root vegetable that grows in the highlands of Peru. It has been a staple food of the local inhabitants for over 2,000 years. Little else grows between 10,000 and 15,000 feet, so it's good that it is highly nutritious.

In fact it's a powerhouse of vital nutrients; chock full of amino acids, vitamins, and minerals. This helps, but the secret appears to be in two of its unique compounds.

Muira puama (*Ptychopetalum olacoides*) is also known as "potency wood" if that gives you an idea of how appreciated it is by both sexes, especially in Brazil.

Chris Killem, aka the Medicine Hunter, has probably done more research on rainforest aphrodisiacs around the world than anyone else. He tells a wonderful story of meeting a Brazilian herbalist who describes how well catuaba and muira puama work together.
http://health.discovery.com/centers/sex/libido/amazon.html

Herbadesiac fun:

- Find a good time for this. That's a really important first step. Next find an aphrodisiac food or aroma that appeals to you. If you have a partner, share. Enjoy your aphrodisiac…

- Check your reaction. Just the act of taking an aphrodisiac can be sexy! Listen inside. Notice how you feel when you take it, taste it or smell it. What changed? If you are with someone ask them what they noticed. That's probably enough right there.

    Just a reminder. This is a natural, gentle process.

Our responses to food or aromas are more likely to come as sighs and whispers than thunder and lightning.

- If you enjoyed this, set some time aside to repeat the 'experiment' using a different aphrodisiac.

- Remember, this is sex we're talking about. It's a big deal! Make it special. Bring in candles. Use scented massage oil. Wear lingerie, and make sure you feel sexy in it. Try something new. Try something crazy for you...toys, maybe? Or sex on the floor! Surprise your partner, surprise yourself.

Aphrodisiacs help. The rest is up to us.

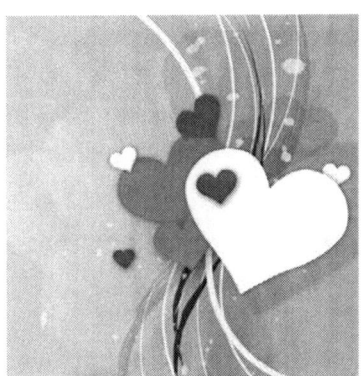

Terra Mar

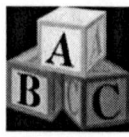 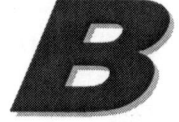 is for Bitters

"Do not worry; eat three square meals a day; say your prayers; be courteous to your creditors; keep your digestion good; exercise; go slow and easy. Maybe there are other things your special case requires to make you happy; but, my friend, these I recommend."
-- **Abraham Lincoln** (1809-1865). 16th U.S. president

What are bitters, and frankly, why would you care? It could be because a) your lover walked out on you and you've got the bitters, b) you ate something that didn't agree with you, your digestion is acting up and wanting bitters, or c) it's freezing cold out and that's giving you the bitters.

Let's go with b), since **B** is for bitters.

Bitters usually refer to a distilled alcoholic drink that has been strongly infused with aromatic herbs, barks, rinds, berries or roots. Bitters taste terrible. They're sharp, unpleasant, and acrid. But that's exactly why they're good for you.

Chinese medicine has a saying about sweet on the tongue being bad for digestion, while bitter on the tongue is healthy for digestion. Roots, tubers, plants and berries are a common part of the diet for those whose daily food is close to the earth, and bitter is a common flavor. For those of us in industrialized countries, bitter has almost entirely disappeared from our modern-day diets.

If it comes across our palettes, our taste buds are shocked. But bitter on the tongue is a great balancer for our entire digestive process.

Bitters are a bit of a cheat sheet. They are easily available, can be great fun as an alcoholic beverage and are good for you as well. They can help mitigate the myriad of weight, nutrition and digestive issues caused by sluggish metabolism.

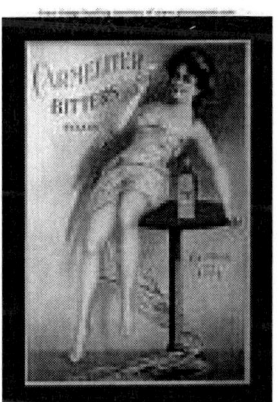

They are a great support in helping us regain lost digestive balance and in tonifying the entire digestive system by helping to stimulate the flow of digestive juices and of bile.

This is key, because if either juices or bile is not flowing well the result can be discomfort, poor digestion, poor nutrient absorption, unnecessary fat storage and bloating. That wouldn't be any body's idea of a good time.

Bitters before, bitters after

Typically bitters are taken as a digestive after a meal to improve digestion or help with upset stomach, but they can also be used as an aperitif to stimulate the appetite.

Well-known bitters in the U.S. include quinine, orange peels, cascarilla, gentian, and angostura bark. You can buy bitters at the grocery. If you're going that route, be careful as a little goes a long way.

I believe the best way to take bitters medicinally is as an alcohol-based tincture. As always, it requires wise and responsible use of herbs.

Most of the bitters mentioned above are from the rainforest and there's a lot more where they came from; the Amazon rainforest has many herbs that are used as bitters. Here are a few of note:

Bitter herbs to play with

Artichoke (*Cynara scolymus*) Humble member of the thistle family, the globe artichoke is pretty amazing. Aside from having an unusual, slightly bitter (and for most of us yummy) flavor it's just plain fun and sexy to eat. The artichoke has been with us for at least 3,000 years, and its culinary attributes are just the beginning.

It is often recommended by herbalists to increase bile production in the liver, increase the flow of bile from the gallbladder, and improve the ability of the bile duct to contract.

These are scientifically proven bile actions, and are typically considered beneficial enough to help in many digestive, gallbladder, and liver disorders.

Moreover, artichoke has gotten a lot of press recently for its exceptionally high levels of antioxidants -- higher than blueberries, chocolate or any other veggie -- and for its cholesterol-lowering effects. It also helps detoxify the liver. In concentrated form it is a prescription medicine in Europe. Humble thistle indeed.

Amargo Bark (*Quassia amara*) Quinine bark, used for malaria and to reduce fever, is one of the rainforest's most famous plants. Centuries before it became known around the world for malaria, it was used as a stomach bitter to treat indigestion and today is used in drinks for the same purpose.

Amargo -- bitter in Spanish -- also goes by the name quassia in the U.S. It is used in the Amazon rainforest like quinine -- for malaria, fevers, and as a digestive. Interestingly, studies have shown amargo bark to be 50 times more bitter than quinine. That puts it somewhere off the charts.

Bitter Melon *(Momordica charantia)* looks like a cucumber or zucchini that got in the way of some radioactive fallout. It is used in the Amazon rainforest as food and as medicine. Though beautiful it may not be, an incredible powerhouse it is.

The whole plant is a wonderful bitter. The leaves and stem are recommended for indigestion and slow digestion, while the fruit is considered helpful for intestinal gas and bloating.

Boldo *(Peumus boldus)* is prescribed in Europe for various gastrointestinal complaints. A sluggish digestive system can result in fermentation where it shouldn't be, followed by bloat, gas, and poor absorption of nutrients.

Boldo is considered one of the best natural remedies for these types of digestive problems by helping stimulate the production and secretion of bile and other digestive juices in the stomach, gallbladder, and liver. If these are working well, the whole digestive process has the potential to function in an optimal way.

Bittertivities:

- Bitter foods include chocolate (minus the sugar of course), bitter melon, olives, citrus peel, brassica veggies, dandelion greens, and escarole. Bitter drinks include coffee, beer, bitters, and quinine.

- How many ways can you find to reintroduce the taste of bitter to your palette?

- Consider picking up a bitter at the store before your next big holiday dinner or big night out. Sip it afterwards. You might be surprised. A wonderful, if

ABC's of Natural Healing

sometimes hard-to-find imported European bitter, is Underberg.

🌿 Check out the ingredients in a few herbal bitters. Recognize anything? Can you make a better-informed decision now as to which you might prefer?

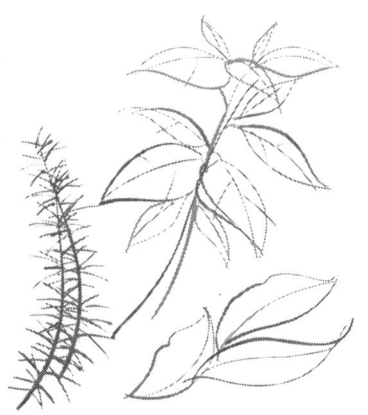

13

Terra Mar

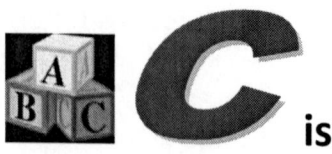 C is for Curanderos

"If you trust Google more than your doctor then maybe it's time to switch doctors." -- **Jadelr and Cristina Cordova,** Chasing Windmills

Curandera is like cure in English. Literally healer. With an 'a' at the end it's female; 'o' instead would be male.

In the broadest definition curanderas and curanderos have been the witches and the druids, the midwives and herbalists, the alchemists, the shamans, the witch doctors and the wise ones. In some form they have been at our sides always. They have been caretakers and healers who have studied in the vast realms of Nature and stepped in as part of a long, unbroken human tradition. They have existed throughout all of human time and in every culture on earth.

In Mayan cultures, and throughout Latin America curanderos are part of a lineage that believes body, mind and spirit are one and that any or all can fall ill. All use natural methods.

Most will pick a specialty and work mainly in that arena. Some specialize in herbs, others massage, others midwifery. All share a belief that healing involves restoring spiritual balance within, and finding balance with Nature and the outer world in which one lives.

If we in the U.S. hear about this long tradition at all, we are most likely to be told that the curandera tradition is witchcraft or quackery. At best, it is considered quaint, local and pretty darn ineffectual.

As North Americans we tend to believe very much in what we can see, feel, touch or prove by scientific method. So for most of us the idea of a curandera as an effective and important healer is quite a stretch. And OMG, our medical establishment, you can imagine what they think. It's a train wreck.

I believe much of the responsibility for stereotyping lies in the education of our medical professionals, which insists on perpetuating a conflict between natural healing and modern medicine. I'll grant there are differences, but they both have validity and it is unproductive to view them as mutually exclusive.

Consider these facts

- All around the world the World Health Organization promotes the use of plants as the number one choice for healing.

- Medicinal plants have been found in the Middle East dating back 60,000 years. Of the eight herbs found, seven are still in use today.

- Today, the primary means of health care for more than 80 percent of the world's population is herbal medicine.

Terra Mar

Meanwhile 300,000 people die each year from over-the-counter and prescription medications *that are properly prescribed and used.*

I bring this up not to discredit western medicine, which has saved my life not once but three times. I bring it up because we tend to have a blind spot and think western medicine is the only, best, or most used form of healing. We even call natural medicine "alternative."

Modern western (allopathic) medicine has an undeniably strong track record in sophisticated surgeries, diagnostics and treatments for cancer and diseases requiring antibiotics.

However if you ask a curandero -- or better yet someone who has been cured by one -- whether their medicine is also powerful, you will hear amazing stories of miracle cures and life-saving interventions.

You'll learn of plants with powerful antibiotic qualities, of plants that reduce fever, counteract venom, close bleeding wounds, heal virulent skin problems, treat depression, calm anxiety, and are successful with cancer and many of the illnesses and conditions treated by western medicine.

Other than treatment methods, another difference of note is interpretation of the root cause of the disturbance. Sometimes allopathic doctors will admit they don't know the origin but can cure the symptom. A curandera may attribute the origin to a shock or fright, to bad air or an evil eye.

Perhaps curanderos would benefit from more openness to western medicine. I am absolutely convinced that we in the U.S. would benefit greatly from being more open not only to the old ways of healing so popular around the world, but to our own homegrown healers -- curanderas and curanderos in our midst.

Curacize yourself:

Expand your thinking about disease

- Think back on your illnesses, accidents, aches, or pains. Pick one and see if you can find a metaphor to explain it. For example, I twisted my ankle and it really hurt – no metaphor there, just swelling and pain. To get to the metaphor what I would look at is this: It happened just as I lunged with one hand to catch the shopping bag that was about to fall out of the car, even though I had my computer in my other hand and the baby right next to me in the stroller. On a hill.

The metaphor: My body is saying SLOW DOWN! Relax. Take a load off your feet. Now see if you can come up with one from your life experience.

Apply the metaphor

- Take the metaphor and imagine yourself right now doing what it is asking. At this level you do not actually have the injury or illness. You are fully healthy, just indulging in the metaphor. In my case, that would be *slowing down*.

- I imagine myself resting, putting my feet up, relaxing, taking time for myself. I imagine this with all my senses, and luxuriate in how good that feels. OK, your turn.

Take yourself by surprise

- Before you leave that pleasant indulgence, set yourself a 'trigger' up to 24 hours in advance. The trigger could be when the sun sets tomorrow, right before going to sleep, or as soon as the kids are in bed. Whatever works for you.

- When your trigger goes off, use great intent and great feeling to once again apply the metaphor. Indulge! Enjoy! Feel yourself healing at a deeper, non-physical level. Savor it.

    You can do this any number of times with the same metaphor. The more often you do it the more powerful it will be for you. Or, you can start with steps 1 – 3 with something else. Remember, it's all good!

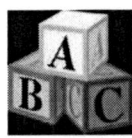 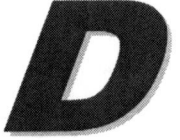 is for Disease

"The art of medicine consists of amusing the patient while nature cures the disease." -- **Voltaire** (French philosopher and author 1694-1778)

Since we'll be talking about disease, let me ask you this: What is ease? What is it for you in your life?

☐   The nice feeling after a good workout

☐   Doing something within your comfort zone

☐   The afterglow of lovemaking

☐   Or? You name one..._____

Whatever it is for you, it's going to involve feelings of well-being and balance. Our bodies, minds, and emotions are constantly seeking balance. When we succeed, we feel healthy. We are at ease. Disease is a disruption in that equilibrium, resulting in an imbalance.

Like a duck to water...

Like ducks appearing calm on the surface while they paddle like crazy under water, our bodies and souls are constantly fending off attacks and bombardments at all levels. You'll find more on this essential life-preserving ability in **I is for Immune, V is for Virus and Y is for Yeast.**

Terra Mar

Our bodies fight microorganisms called pathogens, which attack us armed with seemingly endless variations of nasty bacteria, viruses, protozoa, yeast and fungi.

Similarly, our spirits are under ongoing attack from emotional and verbal abuse, isolation, and a host of social, economic and other life stresses.

At what point is our ease dissed?

Typically we believe we have a disease when we are diagnosed with one. No argument there. But where is the tipping point? After all, the doctor is finding what already exists.

At what point is our ease dissed to the point of disease? Ask a practitioner of Chinese medicine and they'll likely say we are diseased when our energy cannot flow freely through our bodies and causes disruptions.

When we have a disease it is generally a particular organ or a system that is overwhelmed to the point

> "The good physician treats the disease; the great physician treats the patient who has the disease"-- **William Osler** (Canadian Physician, 1849-1919)

it cannot maintain health in balance. Yet we tend to think of our whole selves as sick, having a disease – or worse yet – being the disease. In doctor speak that would be 'the gall bladder in room 43.' For ourselves, it means believing a disease has total power over us.

When I went through cancer several years ago, my naturopath told me something that helped me enormously. It was a profound 'aha' moment for me; one that got me to think differently about cancer and disease in general. Just getting a cancer diagnosis is disempowering, with more assaults likely to follow.

Yet here's what he said:

"How many cells do you have in your body? Fifty or 70 trillion. How many are cancerous? Twenty thousand? Maybe a hundred thousand? You are so much bigger than cancer."

It is true. We are so much bigger than our diseases, even the ones that might kill us. We often give up what a disease can't take – our hope, peace of mind, self-love, and acceptance. There's a lot we have every right to preserve, no matter what.

Here are a few tips that may help:

- **You are huge!** Should you get a disease, and I do mean any, from the common cold to depression and into the major leagues, remember *you are so much bigger than it*. That becomes part of a courage kit, and a positive attitude. They're always good to have handy.

Terra Mar

- 🌿 **Redefine the line between health and disease.** Create a third position that lies between the two: *dis-ease*. When you're feeling great, mark the feeling. Remind yourself how health feels. That way you're more likely to catch the beginnings of the devolution into dis-ease and stop it in its tracks.

- 🌿 **Trust your body to do its best.** Know it constantly wants to help you heal. Set your *mind* to help support your body.

- 🌿 **Let it be!** All three of these pointers entail helping the mind remember. It's amazing how quickly the mind forgets. Imagine, if you can, rain when you are the bright sun, or summer from the depths of winter. That's how hard it is for the mind to imagine health when you are struggling with a disease. Sometimes there's a different way: Let it be and let go! Watch a funny movie, sleep, drink lots of water, and let the battle rage.

Maca.

A great way to stay healthy is to keep your immune system strong. I is devoted to the immune system and you'll find great herbs there.

But I want to bring up maca again here. As you may remember from **A is for Aphrodisiac,** maca is a staple food for people who live high up in the Peruvian Andes and have little access to fruits and vegetables. It is definitely great for the immune system with its large number of nutrients, amino acids, vitamins, and minerals.

No one expects you to eat five pounds of maca a week, but it is readily available here in the States as a valuable supplement to a healthy diet.

Healthytivities:

Identify what ease is for you and write down three moments of balance, comfort and ease.

- Find ways to build what you come up with into your daily routines.

- Identify what puts you into a state of discomfort or unease. Write down at least three of these.

- Find ways to eliminate or minimize them from your life.

- Alternately, if it's something you cannot eliminate or minimize, afterwards find ways to incorporate something from #1 as quickly as possible.

Terra Mar

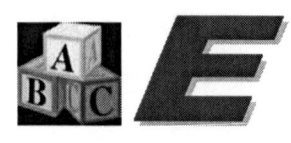

E is for Ethnobotany

"Your body is a temple, but only if you treat it as one."
-- **Astrid Alauda**

Ethnobotany: I'm sure you get the general meaning from the pieces – ethno as in people, from 'ethnos' the Greek word for people. Botany, study of plants. Homo sapiens and flora, a tale as old as time. So ethnobotany is the study of the links between people and plants.

Beyond Science

One could define it more narrowly as the scientific study of how humans use plants, but that's kind of boring. Aside from that, even if you call a cow a horse, it's still a cow. A wish to limit it to 'scientific study' notwithstanding, the interactions between humans and plants transcend categories, including science. Imagine the aroma of a rose, the taste of cinnamon, the sight of a cherry tree in full blossom, or the feel of a soft petal. Now, how would you quantify that?

We humans and plants interact with each other any number of ways that are outside the touch, see, and feel quantifications of science. We teach, learn and re-tell the magical, shamanic, and mais oui, the healing components of plants. There's more. Aromatherapy, plant energetics, incense burning, ceremonials, rituals and gardening are all age-old human plant interactions that may transcend the knowable.

Something I wonder is how shamans and other healers scattered around the world have used the same or similar plants for the same purposes. Rainforests hold literally hundreds of thousands of choices. The answer, depending on your world view, may lie beyond science in the mystical, the coincidental, the logical, the inexplicable, or mythological.

How would a plant feel about that experiment?

Last year Switzerland made an unusual amendment to its constitution. Researchers must now show their proposed study would not undermine the dignity of flora. The regulation followed recommendations by a parliament-appointed panel of philosophers, lawyers, geneticists and theologians.

Yup. It is part of the 'moral consideration of plants for their own sake.' For example, it was decided it would humiliate wheat if humans were to take away its ability to go through its whole life cycle, from seed to seed. That spells no to sterility for Swiss plants, which probably did not make the Swiss office of Monsanto happy.

The deeper question under review is not whether the Swiss have lost their marbles, although many Americans may think so. I think it actually goes beyond the large and thorny (pardon the pun) genetic questions involved. I think the issue here cuts to the core of ethnobotany in its broadest definition.

Exist, persist, and regenerate

Inherent in bringing together a broad coalition of scientists, philosophers, jurists and theologians is the concept that all life matters. I view this amendment as a thinly veiled attempt to ask humans to *consider the sanctity of ALL life.*

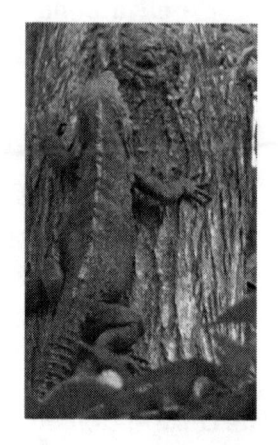

I believe the Swiss are really saying, yes we interact with grains and other flora and it requires that we humans take the moral high ground. It requires stewardship, not manipulation; long-term protections rather than short-term destruction.

Here's another step in the same direction. In September, 2008 the people of Ecuador voted for a new constitution that recognized ecosystem rights as enforceable in a court of law.

Now the nation's rivers, forests and air are no longer mere property, but right-bearing entities with "the right to exist, persist and...regenerate." I just want to repeat – that's *water, air, and flora* that now have constitutional rights in Ecuador.

Ethnobotany holds the potential to blow our minds, expand our horizons and challenge our old constructs. I hope it does. I hope it will help save the planet.

Humans have rights, too

I worked for years at the United Nations. I came in young and flat out starry-eyed. I was awed by the fact that I was in an organization with people from all over the world. I could walk the halls and see native dress from anywhere on earth; I could hear a hodgepodge of languages. Wow, I thought! This is the best of a rainbow coalition. People will come together and achieve amazing results. We can fix world hunger, poverty, human rights abuses and deforestation. For starters.

OK, I already admitted I was starry-eyed, so back off with the kicks and giggles. What I learned in relatively short and shocking order was that we are no better as representatives than we are as individuals.

I also learned that nations are no different than individuals. Just bigger. The crimes and good deeds we do as individuals are simply defended more vociferously and at greater cost by nations.

Whose plant is this anyway?

I fear the same is true for the field of ethnobotany, and in particular for ethnobotanists. There's a flip side to our responsibilities to flora, and it is responsibility to the people who live where we study plants. When ethnobotanists go to the Amazon rainforest to study how indigenous people interact with plants and use them, the same rules of dignity and right to go through their own life processes need apply.

Yet we have witnessed encroachment on ownership and patents, stealing of secrets, interference with rituals and ceremony, disputes over payments for access. Not all these problems are due to greedy, unfeeling northerners. The fact is the experimenter influences the experiment, well-meaning or not. The very presence of ethnobotanists could be construed as cultural interference.

Add in the difficulties of indigenous societies to survive encroachment under the best of circumstances, cultural barriers, economics, politics, environmentalism and more. It is an enormously sensitive and complex arena that needs a great deal of attention.

An egregious example of this is maca. As you already know from **A** and **D**, maca is a staple food in the Amazon highlands. For many centuries it was cultivated and traded by the Indians in exchange for goods they could not grow at altitude.

Enter ethnobotanists who "discover" maca and bring it to the north – and make a small fortune with a patent. In a sophisticated form of biopiracy, large companies identified the plant's active compounds and used them as a basis for a product they patented. This patent was on a plant that had been cultivated and developed for millennia by a people who were receiving no compensation of any kind.

The situation for the local maca growers was improved only when a company came in that believed in giving back to the communities where they did business. A battle ensued for almost a decade. Ultimately companies in Peru were granted free licenses.

This tale is not new. We've seen it in many countries with food, coffee, and other resources. In the case of the rainforest we're not talking about a few plants. Natural plant substances generate more than *$75 billion* in sales each year for the pharmaceutical industry, and an additional $20 billion in herbal supplement sales.

It is in all of our interests that we better understand and research the rainforest's healing plants -but with dignity for flora and human alike.

Ethnercises to play with:

- I've expressed my opinion on the strengths and pitfalls of ethnobotany. What are yours? What about some of your friends, family or colleagues?

- I've also put out that the relations between humans and flora range from the mundane to the mystical. What has your experience been with plants? Does it sound odd, or have you had any plant interactions you'd like to discuss? Email me at **terra@oneplanetherbs.com** if you have any thoughts you'd like to share.

🌿 Finally, if you're willing to stretch, search out a plant, bush or tree you find especially beautiful. When nobody is looking, see what happens when you tell it (telepathically) how you feel. Does it respond with a small movement? Do you have any sensation? Do you hear a response?

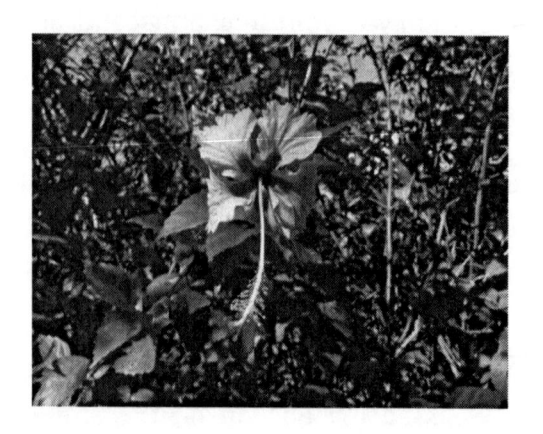

F is for Fatigue

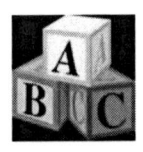

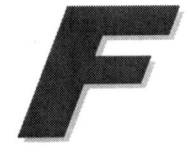

"Our own physical body possesses a wisdom which we who inhabit the body lack. We give it orders which make no sense." -- **Henry Miller**, American novelist (1891 – 1980)

Don't you just hate it when the very thought of doing something makes you tired? Especially if it's not eleven o'clock at night!

Our bodies have their own natural rhythms and that's all good. Fatigue and flat out exhaustion are fine after we've done a strenuous hike, been on the run hour after hour, or done things that wipe us out. I'm female, but going clothes shopping wipes me out faster than anything I can think of! As long as you know what's causing the fatigue that's fine. And that's the kind of fatigue I'm dealing with here.

I'm talking about natural fatigue that is stress-induced either because you've done too much physical or mental work or because you're, well... stressed. Stress is exhausting.

What I'm *not* talking about is fatigue that you're not familiar with, that is consistent and impinging on your life style or fatigue that has you concerned. Those may all be related to medical conditions and as you already know if you have any health questions, see your doctor or health care practitioner. Nothing in this book is intended to diagnose, treat or cure any illness; this is all for information only. With that caveat in place:

What do you do about fatigue?

That depends. There are different reasons for exhaustion or fatigue. A, B, or C...

A: Is it late and you're still trying to work?

In that case go to bed and sleep. Whatever it is you're working on or playing with, you'll do better when you're refreshed. I'm a night owl and often want to push the envelope though I'll pay a price the next day.

Our bodies give us messages in layers from gentle taps to wallops. I find it best to heed the early signs and avoid getting hit upside the head. I sometimes need to be my own parent and tell myself to stop what I'm doing and go to bed!

Here are two of my favorite bed time helpers:

Mulungu (*Erythrina mulungu*) Mulungu is deeply calming, and has been used for centuries as a natural sedative and to treat anxiety. In a 2003 study in Brazil, scientists found it worked in a similar way to diazepam, a well-known anti-anxiety pharmaceutical drug.

Passionflower aka **maracuja** (*Passiflora incarnata*): Unlike many other rainforest herbs, passionflower is actually well-known here for its health benefits, delicious fruit and beautiful flower. It has been used for at least 400 years as an herbal medicine. It is recommended to calm and tone the nerves, promote relaxation, combat sleep problems and insomnia, and treat pain.

B: Are you exhausted because you're coming up on a deadline?

Is it finals week? Are you busy working on a complex project? Are you on a collision course with a deadline? If so, that's a different story altogether. In that case I would suggest you consider some of the following rainforest herbs. They all support healthy energy.

Before I list them, I want to explain that these herbs do not contain caffeine or anything that sends your system into an "upper."

It's an entirely different concept of energy from Red Bull or a cup a jo. No jitters. No high. Rather than stimulating, these herbs support, tonify, balance, and soothe the central nervous system. They help the body find proper balance. The result is vastly improved focus through a deep and solid energy.

Jatobá (*Hymenaea courbaril*) is in a category of its own for healthy, long-lasting energy. (**see J is for Jatobá**) It works as a natural energy tonic that supports the central nervous system and tones and balances overall body functions. It is a wonderful, helpful natural remedy for fatigue.

Chuchuhuasi (*Maytenus krukovii*) Like many rainforest herbs, chuchuhuasi has many uses. An enormous canopy tree, its bark has been used medicinally for centuries. It is a great antidote to fatigue and helps with aches and pains as well. Chuchuhuasi is sometimes referred to as 'go juice' and is served as a drink both for locals and tourists who are about to go trekking in the rainforest.

Sarsaparilla (*Smilax officinalis*) falls into an especially important category of herbs known as 'adaptogenic.' An adaptogen works in ways science has yet to understand to bring an organ or a system into balance. Sarsaparilla root is a tonic that helps fight fatigue and returns a healthy energy by toning, balancing, and strengthening body functions.

Catuaba. As I noted in **A is for Aphrodisiac**, aside from its other benefits catuaba is great for a pleasant night's sleep. This rainforest herb is gaining recognition in the U.S. now, but it has been highly valued for ages in the rainforest. It is calming, reduces anxiety and is healthy for the central nervous system.

Or C: are you coping with high levels of stress that are going to last for a while?

This could be things like money troubles, a layoff, increased expenses or declining income. It could be legal issues, relationship trouble, having your kids hit the teen years. You see where I'm going with this. This a third reason for fatigue, and while the herbs above are good, exhaustion from this long-term stress needs immune builders as well. Chuchuhuasi and sarsaparilla are particularly good for the immune system. But here's another one.

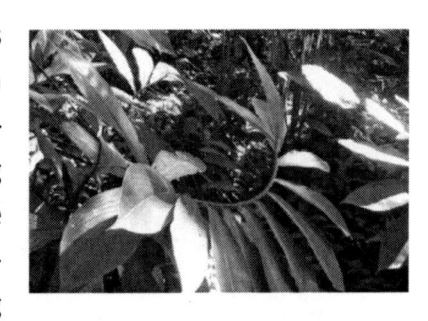

Cat's claw aka **uña de gato** (*Uncaria tomentosa*) Cat's claw is considered a powerful immune booster, and I say a lot more about it in **I is for Immune**. Decades of research have provided scientific explanations for this plant's popularity. Even Dr. John Bastyr, namesake for the University, often referenced it as a tonic.

A friend of mine who leads trips to Peru makes sure he builds in time for the market so he can stock up on cat's claw for use as a daily tonic once he's back in the States.

Terra Mar

Fatiguebuster activities:

- Lifestyle is always the first line of remedy. Take time to think about your own level of fatigue and exhaustion (physical and emotional) and explore what brings it on.

- Next look at your Mon – Fri week. What exhausts you most about it? Pick only the top one.

- Now fill in the blank: _____ wears me out and utterly exhausts me.

- How can you fix that? Get rid of it? Lessen it? Write down your answer: As of today I am going to lessen the impact of this by _____
_____

Note to self: in exactly one week from today I'm going to check back and see how I feel.

- When you check back, if you feel you have made changes, give yourself a big *Better Health Gold Star Award*. Then feel free to add another one and do the same thing.

  If you do two or three of these and make the needed changes I promise you *will* feel it in better health, less fatigue, more energy and more FUN!

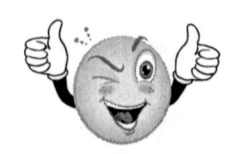

G is for Gaia

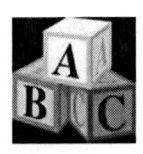

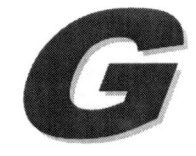

"Deep in the heart of the infinite darkness, a tiny blue marble goes whirling through space. Born in the splendor of God's holy vision, sliding along like a tear down His face. Look closer, you'll see the whole wide holy wonder of oceans and mountains, rivers and trees. And the strangest creation of many, the human, a creature of laughter, freedom and dreams" -- **Kris Kristofferson**

Gaia and imbalance

The derivation of Gaia is from two stems in Greek -- ge for earth (as in geology) and aia: grandmother (who knew?). Grandmother Earth. She was revered as the primal Goddess, She who began life. Gaia personified creator of Earth out of Chaos. I was pleased, and duly humbled, to learn her Roman name was Terra.

The name Gaia has increased in popularity in the past few decades due not only to the Hypothesis, but due to New Agers as well. There are bookstores, groups, Mother Earth images and much more that carry the name Gaia. Often the New Age approach ascribes a consciousness to Gaia that was not in the Hypothesis.

The man who developed the Gaia Hypothesis was more of a muggle than a New Ager. James Lovelock was a scientist who was working on a project for NASA at the time his ideas began to take shape in the 1960's.

His assignment was to develop experiments for detecting life on Mars. He ended up annoying his employer big time because NASA was seeking any rationale to land a rover on the planet. Instead Lovelock argued that he was certain no life existed on Mars because it was in a state of what he called 'dead equilibrium.' His interests began to wander to the opposite of that.

He became intrigued by the fact that unlike other planets in our solar system, the atmosphere of our "tiny blue marble" was in a state he described as 'far from equilibrium.' It was a unique condition that remained constant and supported life.

From this he posited that a complex process was keeping our planet in this unlikely state of life-supporting imbalance.

The science behind it is complex and pretty fascinating, but no worries. I couldn't explain it if I wanted to. For our purposes it is enough to know that it has been looked at, experimented with, tested and worked on for decades. Despite its share of critics and naysayers, it turns out that Lovelock's improbable hypothesis has been supported by a number of scientific experiments and has provided many useful predictions.

Because of this, the Hypothesis graduated to a Theory, and is now properly referred to as the Gaia Theory.

ABC's of Natural Healing

OK, you may say. But what the bleep does this have to do with herbs, health, and the rainforest?

Much more than would be apparent at first blush. Current scientific thinking poses a 'weak' and a 'strong' Gaia theory. There is overwhelming agreement in the scientific community on the basics, or 'weak' theory.

Part of it is that we humans are making huge changes in the longstanding balance of nature and that the entire planet and all its inhabitants are impacted by the ensuing regulation that is taking place.

In 2006, Lovelock came out with a new book: *"The Revenge of Gaia: Why the earth is fighting back - and how we can still save humanity."* In it he points specifically to the damage we have done to the rainforests and the resultant loss of planetary biodiversity.

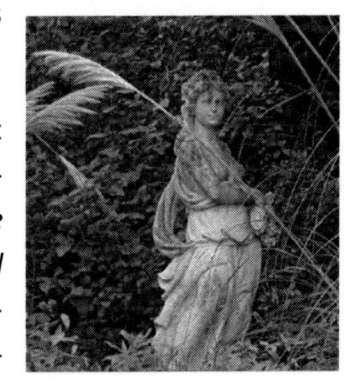

Lovelock maintains that the lack of respect we have shown Earth is testing Gaia's capacity to minimize the effects of additional greenhouse gases in the atmosphere.

Once we accept the now commonplace notion that human activities impact the biosphere, atmosphere, seas and land, we take on both consciousness and responsibility. In a way it's odd because we are burdened with responsibility for what we cannot possibly fully comprehend: the future impacts of our current activities on all of life. And that, it turns out, is the heart of the problem.

Often in discussions of climate change and acidification of the oceans we make the assumption that if unchecked our actions will destroy the planet. According to the Gaia Theory however, that is not so. Gaia supports life, just not necessarily life as we may know or want it. We may not be 'destroying' our planet at all, simply creating new conditions that could make life for future generations anywhere from intolerable to uninhabitable.

Agree or disagree with the Gaia Theory, it is still of value because it raises questions that are as critical as they are unpleasant.

What we are experiencing now is the beginning of our uncertain legacy to future generations.

Consider these three results of the Gaia Theory:

- *It broadens the discussion of human impacts.* We tend to think in straight lines -- we cut some trees, pave over the earth and get a parking lot. Simple. Cause, effect. Action, result. The problem is that our impacts are often unseen, long-term, completely unpredictable, and ripple out in complex ways that do not fit our linear thinking.

Anything that encourages us to take pause and seek better stewardship of our planet is beneficial as far as I'm concerned.

- *It raises the specter of life as we wouldn't want to know it.* It elevates the discussion about consequences beyond simply 'we're ruining the planet.' It suggests that our actions could have consequences that would not destroy the planet, but rather create conditions in which human life and other forms of life we need to sustain us are not supported.

- *It creates a sense of urgency.* While the Gaia Theory does not try to quantify the pace of change, it has opened a serious discussion about the probability of human-driven *irreversible* damage. This is worse than talking about life insurance or a will. This is the verbal and scientific equivalent of a root canal, but no less important for the pain.

Indigenous societies and Gaia

A few short centuries ago North America was the battleground for survival of indigenous cultures. As North America's First People's lands were taken away, their numbers declined and they were almost destroyed, along with their traditional ways. So it is today in the rainforests of South America.

Terra Mar

In 1500 there were between six and nine million indigenous people in the rainforests of Brazil. Today, fewer than 250,000 inhabitants survive. (The Nature Conservancy) Still the destruction continues. Today a full twenty percent of the rainforest is gone, with dire predictions for the coming years.

We certainly cannot blame the local inhabitants who raze the land. Starvation is a strong driver. Besides, this destruction runs completely counter to Earth-bound cultures. It is a form of cultural suicide.

Indigenous societies have not needed a Gaia Theory to determine or temper their interactions with the Earth. Traditionally Earth-based cultures never felt they had a right to change the world around them or to take on nature.

Instead indigenous cultures tend to see themselves, animals, rivers, oceans and plants as inextricable and intrinsic parts of nature. Harming any part harms them.

Indigenous cultures generally have many Gods and Goddesses and a rich tradition of myth and folk tales. If you believe all of life is woven of the same fabric it is easy to view all beings that inhabit the Earth and all the places they inhabit – land, air, water, forest, desert and mountains as interdependent.

Even the line between animate and inanimate objects becomes blurred because the world is alive. Knowledge and wisdom is developed not outside or above nature, but from observations, interactions and closeness with nature.

My point on the Gaia Theory is this. Knowledge is power. But so is action. We don't have a definitive answer on the Gaia Theory, but we know both knowledge and action, and dare I add ancient wisdom are desperately needed right now.

I would rather err on the side that supports life and stewardship and assume you would as well. I am merely offering you another arrow in your quiver.

I think it only fitting that I let Mr. Lovelock have the last word:

"You may find it hard to swallow the notion that anything as large and apparently inanimate as the Earth is alive. Surely, you may say, the Earth is almost wholly rock, and nearly all incandescent with heat.

The difficulty can be lessened if you let the image of a giant redwood tree enter your mind. The tree undoubtedly is alive, yet 99% of it is dead.

The great tree is an ancient spire of dead wood, made of lignin and cellulose by the ancestors of the thin layer of living cells which constitute its bark.

Terra Mar

How like the Earth, and more so when we realize that many of the atoms of the rocks far down into the magma were once part of the ancestral life of which we all have come. "
-- ***The Ages of Gaia*** by James Lovelock, 1988

Gaiacizes:

- Consider the three discussion points on the Gaia Theory. What is your belief? Talk about them with friends as you seek clarity in your own mind.

- Is any of this a call to action for you?

- Do you believe that with such overwhelming challenges anything you may do would matter?

- If your answer is yes, what can you do different tomorrow from what you did yesterday?

- If your answer is no, could you accept that with so much at stake it might still be better to try?

H is for Herbs

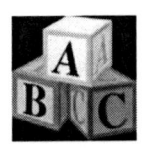

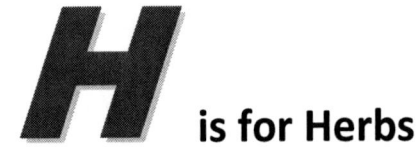

"The most beautiful thing we can experience is the mysterious. It is the source of all art and science."
-- Albert Einstein

Some of you may be tempted to skip over **H** because you're already sold on the value of herbs. I'm making it easy by bolding each point. There's always something new to learn, so peruse, scan or read at will.

One of my first encounters with the power of herbs was with healing clay. I was barely 20 and training several hours a day outside at a martial arts camp in the woods of Washington. We were all barefoot. Well over a hundred people and I was the one to step on an old nail. It broke the skin, but I kept training. By evening my foot was infected.

A friend brought me some green French healing clay, which to my untrained eye just looked like more dirt, the stuff that had infected my foot. She was convincing though, so I tried it. By morning the infection was gone. I thought, now that's a coincidence. My foot healed even though I used that stuff. I had my world view and it didn't include green goop healing my foot. I saw no reason to use it again, despite my friend's instructions.

Terra Mar

By lunch my foot was getting worse, by late afternoon it was infected again. This really surprised me because I thought I had healed. Since I had nothing else around (and my friend insisted) I put on the messy goop again. I was honestly afraid it would make my foot worse, but within a few hours the infection was gone.

Was I convinced? Of course not. It took another two times of the same game for me to really believe it was the clay that was taking away the infection. After that shake-up to my universe, trying herbs was an easy next step.

The five most important things you need to know about herbs

1: Parsley and basil are not herbs. Just kidding. Parsley and basil *are* herbs, but they're not the *only* herbs. Often people think an herb has to be a small bushy-like plant. Not so. In herbal medicine, *any* plant or part of a plant can be used to benefit health.

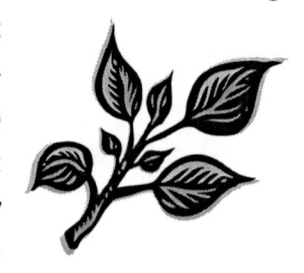

This includes flowers, bushes, vines and trees, even huge rainforest canopy trees. Ginger root, aloe cactus leaves, bark of the huge rainforest tree pau d'arco, and elder berries all are used for therapeutic purposes and qualify as "herbs." More than 2,000 herbs are used medicinally today.

The biodiversity of the rainforest is so enormous that *less than one percent of its millions of species have been studied by scientists for their healing potential.* (The Nature Conservancy) As to an actual number, science hasn't figured that one out yet. Estimates range from two million to a hundred million.

Speaking of which, have I already mentioned that according to the Nature Conservancy scientists also estimate we lose over 137 species of plants and animals every day through rainforest deforestation? While I'm on sad factoids I'll add that we are talking about an ecosystem that is at least 55 million years old, (Wikipedia), covers a mere two percent of the earth's surface yet supports over half our planet's wild plants, trees and wildlife. (Mongabay.com) And we continue to destroy it. Go figure.

2: Herbs have been safely used for thousands of years to improve health, cure wounds of all kinds and heal disease. Cultures all over the world have gathered a vast body of knowledge regarding the power of herbs to create and support improved health. Much of this information has been passed down to us through Western herbalism, Ayurvedic herbalism, and Chinese Medicine. There's more on this in **R is for Remedies**.

As I mentioned earlier, 80% of the world's population still uses herbal remedies as their primary health care. Indigenous cultures continue to pass along invaluable herbal knowledge from one generation to the next. It

Terra Mar

includes which parts of plants are beneficial and how to prepare them; whether to boil, steep, or crush, how long to use and in what quantities to access the plant's medicinal properties.

Sadly, as tribes disappear and remaining inhabitants assimilate, much of this specialized knowledge is being lost. There are some wonderful programs to support the passing of the torch from one generation to the next. These are critically important for us all.

3. Herbs are used to improve almost any area of health. This includes everything from mood swings to blood pressure, from exhaustion to lactation. Furthermore, one herb is frequently used for apparently unrelated health issues. This is quite different from the targeted pharmaceuticals of western medicine.

For example, aloe vera gel is used to heal sunburn and cleanse the digestive system; bitter melon treats malaria and snake bite. Cat's claw has been used to treat tumors and the flu. Chanca piedra, or "stone breaker," is a common remedy for kidney stones and diabetes.

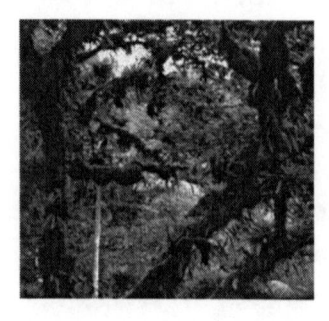

4. Many of our prescription drugs are based on herbal substances. For example, ephedra is an herb that has long been used in Chinese herbology to treat respiratory problems. Ephedrine is the active ingredient in ephedra, and ephedrine is the basis for many pharmaceutical products medicating asthma and other respiratory problems. In addition, approximately 25 percent of prescription drugs in use today have an herbal component. Many of our cancer, heart, and other wonder drugs are originally from herbs, mostly rainforest herbs.

5. Herbs are safe. But don't confuse safe with harmless. Bread, chicken, and mushrooms are also safe—if the bread is not moldy, the chicken is not spoiled, and the mushrooms are not gathered ignorantly off the forest floor. When we take herbal supplements, we need to know what we're doing. Some herbal remedies may interfere with prescription drugs or intensify their impact. This doesn't mean herbs are dangerous—it just means they do in fact, affect our bodies. Since we take herbs to help us heal, that's a good thing.

Just remember to do your research and proceed responsibly. Talk to your health care professional. Taken properly and used responsibly, herbs just may help you feel better than you ever imagined.

Herbs to play with:

I think it's time to try some hands-on herb fun. The simplest way to enjoy herbs, other than tea or aromatherapy, is in the bath.

Terra Mar

Here are a few fun ways:

- Put a large handful of herbs into an enamel pot, cover with water, and bring to a boil. Reduce the heat and let simmer for about 20 minutes. Strain and pour the liquid into the bath. Any mix of your favorites should do it. Enjoy the soak for 20 – 30 minutes.

- Gather the leftover herbs into a muslin bag and them use as a scrub.

- Create an herbal bath sachet. Get some muslin, easily available at Joann's or other crafts store and some string. You could also use thin cotton from a worn out sheet. Put the herbs into the muslin bag, tie it and attach it to the faucet so the hot water runs through it. You could also use a tea infuser. You won't be able to use quite as much of the herbs, but it comes with a chain so it's an easy attachment to the faucet.

- You could also combine the methods. Place the muslin bag into boiling water, let it simmer a bit and then dump the whole thing – bag and liquid into the tub. Yum. Best of both worlds. Make sure you scrub with the bag and rinse with the liquid. Indulge and enjoy!

- For herbs you're likely to have around or to which you're likely to have easy access you could use a mix of what appeals -- lavender, orange or lemon peels (organic only please), rose petals, geranium flowers, German chamomile, mint, rosemary, sage, nutmeg, thyme, eucalyptus, or any others you are comfortable with and that match your sensory standards.

- If you want to take this a step further, you can easily research which scents work well together for a particular result -- as in aromatherapy. Some will be more relaxing, others more stimulating, and so on.

- A great place to start is with herbalist and herb teacher par excellence, John Gallagher at Learning Herbs: http://www.learningherbs.com/.

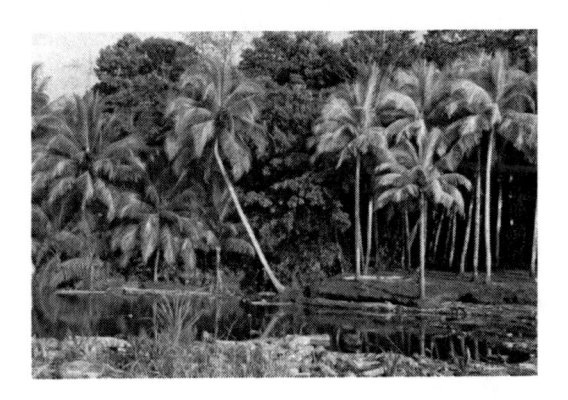

Terra Mar

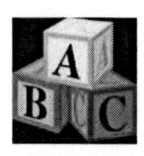

is for Immune

"A child who is protected from all controversial ideas is as vulnerable as a child who is protected from every germ. The infection, when it comes- and it will come - may overwhelm the system, be it the immune system or the belief system." – **Jane Smiley** (Pulitzer Prize-winning author)

I'm grateful for 'I' because it gives me the chance to highlight one of my personal faves among these wonderful helping plants. As you know by now, the pharmacopeia of rainforest herbs is humungous. Still, as in the night sky where you find a star that sets the gold standard for bright, so too with rainforest herbs. Later in this chapter I'll let the light stream out, but let's first take a look at what immune support herbs are supporting.

Oh Toxic World, You Won't Get Me

There is general agreement that the world is a far more toxic place than it used to was. More chemicals and toxins are in the air, in the earth, in the seas, and, of course in us.

The Natural Step (www.naturalstep.org) is a science-based approach out of Sweden that provides guiding principles for living within the resources of our planet. I took a seminar on TNS and they passed around a sheet of paper filled with the results of a chemical analysis. It was a long list and looked pretty bad. Then they asked us to guess what it was. Nobody got the right answer.

The nasty assortment of unpronounceable chemicals was trace elements in women's breast milk. In one recent study, a quarter of the women's milk was so toxic that had it been formula it would have been pulled from the shelves. We have more toxins in us than our parents did and our children are likely to have more than we do.

It's not as if we didn't always need our immune systems to function well; our immune system is at least as important to life as air in our lungs or a beating heart. It's just that in the toxic 21st we're attacked more, which means our immune systems are working harder than ever before. Overall we are living longer so our immune systems need to work not only *harder* but *longer* as well.

What's the immune system anyway?

Excluding viruses, which may not be life forms anyway, **(see V is for Virus)** all living things have some means of protecting themselves from attack. No functional immune system, no life. Some may not even be complex enough to be called a system while ours is a highly refined network. All have the same basic protective functions.

Terra Mar

We know human body systems are complex, but other pale by comparison with the intricacies of our immune system. It's really quite the do. I'd go so far as to say if our immune system were a movie actor, it might not look as good as Brad or Angelina, but would definitely walk away with the Oscar.

It is an astoundingly 'intelligent' network of biological processes that protects us by identifying and killing pathogens that cause disease, and tumor cells that destroy healthy ones. The system is comprised of various types of proteins, cells, organs, and tissues, all of which interact in an elaborate and dynamic dance.

Its Sherlock Holmsian detection capabilities cover everything from bacteria, parasites and microbes to viruses and toxins. It's our own private army working 24/7 to protect us from outside invasion.

Corpuscles and corpses

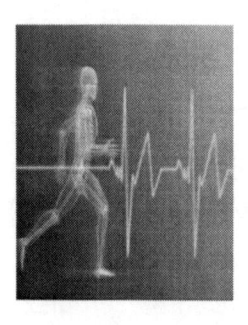

To get an idea of how much invades us, consider the common corpse. Once we no longer have an immune system to protect us, we devolve *sometimes in a matter of hours* into finger food for animals much lower down the food chain. Within weeks, we're bones. The only reason this doesn't happen while we're alive is our immune system.

Detection is not as easy as you may think, Watson. Not only can pathogens evolve quickly, but they're not stupid and they don't want to die so they try to hide from our immune system's detectors. Even once it locates the intruder, our system needs to stay on the alert. It has the all-important job of making sure it's got a real intruder, which can be a great impersonator of our own healthy cells and tissues.

Our immune systems also need to remember pathogens or we would forever be getting colds, viruses and all the stuff kids get. As we grow up our immune system helps us adapt by remembering. It allows us to make use of vaccinations, stops us from getting the same illnesses repeatedly, and helps us stay healthy longer.

Smile: Your T Cells are Watching

I have to put in a word about one part of the system called T Cells. I'm personally indebted to mine because they helped get rid of the cancer that thought it could get away with murder. My T(ough) guys showed them who was the boss of me. I also think they're totally cool because you can increase the number of T Cells in your body through exercise or by being happy. Go ahead and laugh -- it's healthy and your T Cells love it, but it's true.

On the other hand, you don't even want to know all the ways things can go wrong. There are all the autoimmune illnesses, there's genetically induced weakness in immune function, age-induced weakness, overactive immune reaction causing allergies, and of course, sadly, there's AIDS which, as a reminder, is an acronym for *Acquired Immune Deficiency Syndrome*.

Despite the long laundry list, for most of us, for most of our lives our immune systems are the humble, secret, but brightest of stars that keep us shining from the inside out. Now that's worth protecting!

Speaking of Stars:

Immune *modulators* adjust (or modulate) the functioning of the immune system as a whole. Immune *stimulants* promote increased activity or production of immune cells. In that sense exercise or happiness are immune stimulants. **Cat's claw (F is for Fatigue)** is both an immune modulator and an immune stimulant.

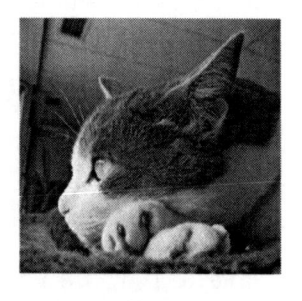

It belongs to that elite group of adaptogen herbs. Science hasn't figured how yet, but in some ways these plants restore the normal functions of an organ or a system, whichever direction it needs to find balance.

Cat's claw has gotten some press in the U.S. as a support for patients going through chemo and is commonly used recommended by herbalists for chronic fatigue

ABC's of Natural Healing

syndrome, depression, lupus, inflammatory conditions, and intestinal disorders. One of the amazing things about cat's claw is that it rises to the top of the list for all the ills it helps.

Research has been ongoing since the 1970's and science is validating many of its attributes. Some years ago in an article in New Life magazine, cat's claw was described as having so many therapeutic uses that it far surpassed such well known botanicals as **echinacea, golden seal, astragalus, Siberian ginseng, and even reishi and shitake mushrooms.**

In my book, oh, this is my book. Anyway, in my world, it's a requirement for cold and flu season, also when travelling or in any other situation where you're exposed to unfamiliar or many germs, bacteria or toxins. It's also safe enough to be used as a daily tonic.

Immunercizes:

- Other fabulous immune builders from the Amazon rainforest include **pau d'arco, samambaia, and bitter melon.** Consider researching these. You may be amazed at how much they do. If you're on the web, start with Raintree Nutrition at www.raintree.com for a thorough science-based review.

- Are you one of those people who gets a bug from recycled airplane air? If so, remembering the disclaimers about using herbs, consider taking some cat's claw before you fly and see if it makes a difference for you. I'd love to hear your stories. Just email me at terra@oneplanetherbs.com.

🌿 A client of mine told me she used cat's claw for a gum problem, and her pain was gone in 30 minutes. She didn't know it was an anti-inflammatory, but thought it might help her immune system fight off the infection.

🌿 Thank your immune system. You can do this by adding some extra physical activity into your day, adding one food to your diet that is high in anti-oxidants and nutrient-rich. And you can also just say thank you immune system! If you're so inclined.

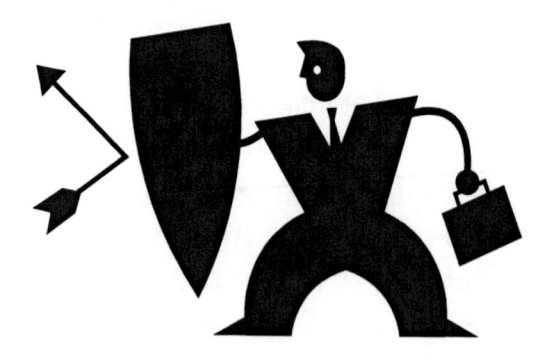

J is for Jatobá

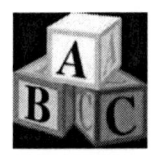

"You can observe a lot just by watching."-- **Yogi Berra** (considered the greatest baseball catcher of all time)

When I began playing with rainforest herbs one of my first acts was to get my hands on **jatobá** (*Hymenaea courbaril*). Since you use the bark, it needs to be boiled to bring out its healing qualities. It's a small effort for a great deal in return.

I had been offered it as a drink in Brazil. I loved its earthy flavor and found it gave me a fabulous energy that I couldn't quite describe at first. I couldn't describe it because even though I'd had ginseng and other herbal tonic teas I responded to jatobá in a way that was new for me.

It was like speed, except without the speed. Not clear? OK, it felt like a boost to my cognitive abilities. I could focus better and longer without any of the feel of a caffeinated drink. Since I knew it had no caffeine I took it in the evening. A mistake I made only once.

I tend to be a night owl even when I have to get up early the next day. So I was pretty bleary-eyed the next morning, having finally gone to bed in the wee hours. My Brazilian hosts got a kick out of it. People in that part of the world know that if you want to sleep before

Terra Mar

midnight you don't drink jatobá in the evening. The energy it gives can last up to to seven hours.

Don't be fooled. Use good wood

What I didn't know about jatobá was that it is the beautiful Brazilian Cherry wood used as flooring. It's not actually in the cherry family. It's "big leaf" mahogany, a canopy rainforest hardwood that is in serious trouble.

It takes around 60 years for the tree to mature and it can reach a height of 500 feet. Often referred to as "green gold," one mahogany tree can net up to $130,000 in furniture.

The temptation has lured illegal loggers, with the result that the trees are severely endangered. Due in large part to the work of Greenpeace, the U.S., the world's largest importer of mahogany, agreed to add jatobá to a convention that requires permits, proof of documentation, and proof that the shipment is not harming the survival of the species.

If you are interested in the wood, make sure you check that it has been certified through the Forest Stewardship Council. You will see **"FSC Certified"** displayed prominently, otherwise it is not FSC-certified.

That certification was set up in the early 1990's in a collaborative effort between environmental organizations and timber companies. There are other certifications, but none of them are as valuable. FSC is the gold standard.

The mighty mahogany is good for many things -- other than being illegally slaughtered. Jatobá is not only of value as a canopy tree that protects animal life and other plants, it is contains amazing healing properties in its own right.

Its popularity doesn't have to be its downfall as has happened with other healing plants. We can continue to use it for the valuable wood that it is while protecting it for all of us, present and future generations, and benefit from the many attributes it offers as a living being.

Obviously it is a great tonic. It is also used to treat urinary tract infections, yeast and fungal infections, and nail fungus, The copal resin at the base of the tree is delightfully aromatic. It is dug up and burned as incense. Its fruit is edible but nicknamed "stinky toe" to describe its taste and smell.

An undocumented use

I have an electric toothbrush and sometimes get a little obsessive about the gunk that accumulates around and under the holder. It's kind of a pain to clean since the inside part has little rings that are hard to get at.

One day in a flash of brilliance I decided to use a solution of jatobá mixed with a little water and vinegar.

Terra Mar

Worked like a charm. I figured if I could just find a way to make the jatobá colorless I could market it as a household cleaner and give muscle-bound Mr. Clean something to cross his big arms about.

Herb fun:

- Do you have a favorite herb? Doesn't have to be from the rainforest. If you have one, Google it and find out its properties. Then try something with it you haven't done before – like gargling with chamomile or making a lavender rinse. Be creative. Have fun. I'd love to hear what you come up with.

- Check out your local flooring store to see if they carry Brazilian Cherry, which they probably do. Ask them if it's FSC-certified. Consider a letter, email or phone call to the buyer explaining why it's important, or a note of thanks if they got it right.

- Bring a little more Nature to your doorstep. Every time we bring nature closer, we connect with life's web. It helps us remember how important a robust ecosystem is to us humans. That's only good.

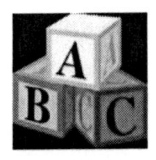

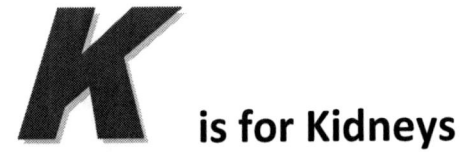

"And in the end it's not the years in your life that count. It's the life in your years." -- **Abraham Lincoln**

King Kidney

Though they resemble a humble bean or large earlobe, Kidney is King. They come in pairs and ideally you want both functioning very well. We're mostly water and they regulate our body's water levels. They also perform a critical clean-up function for us by removing waste products from our blood.

My father used to tell a joke about a boy who wasn't particularly bright. When asked about the placement of the stomach, lungs, heart and intestines he got them all correct. The teacher complimented him and in response the boy nodded, pointed to his forehead and said, "Yeah, kidneys."

I still find it hard to picture where kidneys are without the dumb joke coming to mind. To help us both out I've included an anatomically correct picture.

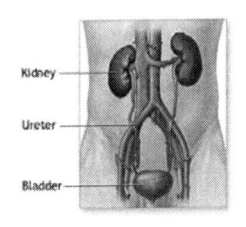

Chinese take on Kidney

In old Chinese medical theory organs refer to functionality rather than a physical organ. Each is a mini system of sorts and has physiological, emotional and spiritual aspects. For example, Kidney (as opposed to the western kidney organ with a small k) is related to fear at the emotional level, water more functionally, and with the origin of life at the spiritual level.

The kidneys are believed to be the repository for our original Essence (Jing). The theory goes that each of us is born with a supply of qi, élan, energy, pizzazz, call it what you will. Kidney, root of everything, stores that for us. We can add to this prenatal energy through healthy life style, and that too is stored in the Kidney.

In both this very old system and also in our relatively new western view, the kidneys are a source of healthy life. Kidney is King; therefore we not only want our kidneys to work well. We want them to do it with as little stress as possible.

The most common problem with kidneys is stones. This extremely painful condition afflicts over five percent of the population. Each year people make almost 3 million kidney stone-related visits to health care providers, and more than a half million people go to the ER for kidney stone problems!

Most times patients will get pain medication and be sent home to drink lots of water. The best preventive care is to drink lots of water, which shouldn't be too difficult. Yeah, right.

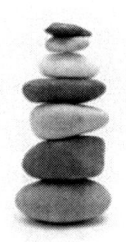

Enter chanca piedra

If you want to support your friendly, hardworking kidneys you could try a rainforest plant that's now getting a lot of attention in the U.S. It's got an unusual two-word name, but that's because the word Chanca is from the Quechua, an indigenous language in S. America, meaning 'to break.' (See Q is for Quechua). Piedra will be more recognizable for 'stone' if you speak Spanish.

Chanca Piedra (*Phyllanthus niruri*) = Break-stone, or in slightly more sensible English, stone breaker. The stones it refers to are the ones we don't want either in the gallbladder or the kidneys. Chanca piedra, also translated as shatter-stone, seems to break or shatter the stones into small pieces and they are then passed out of the body.

Since the 1960's there have been at least 300 studies on chanca piedra. Findings indicate it supports the kidneys, gallbladder, bladder and liver, relieves pain, reduces sugar in the blood and helps lower cholesterol and blood pressure.

Chanca piedra studies have also indicated it has antiviral properties against Hepatitis B and HIV. This web site has an in-depth article on it:
http://www.herballegacy.com/Chanca_Piedra_Thomas.html

One of the best aspects of chanca piedra is that in all the studies and various uses no one is reporting toxicity in any of the clinical studies.

The only side effect is an occasional case of the cramps as stones are expelled.

Given the pain of kidney and gall stones, I find it particularly interesting that a strong pain relieving component has also been discovered in the chanca piedra family. When it comes to inflammatory pain, it tested three times stronger than morphine.

The list of traditional uses is long and mighty.

Epilogue

The Way of the Peaceful Warrior, the first book by Dan Millman, (made into a movie some years back) takes place when Millman was a professional gymnast at UC Berkeley. He meets his guru, an elderly gas station attendant named Socrates.

One of my favorite moments in the book was where Soc challenges Millman to a competition in which they would show each other their best move. This delighted Millman who jumped on a table and performed a dazzling gymnastic display. More than a little proud of himself, he waits for Soc's countermoves.

Instead, Soc goes into the bathroom, comes out with a glass of water and for his best move, drinks it. When Soc claims victory and Millman goes nuts, Soc calmly explains that his kidneys told him he needed water and asks Millman if he can hear his body like that.

Kidneycises:

- Did you know your kidneys will stop putting out thirst signals if you don't pay attention to the feeling of thirst?

- For one day, drink extra water and listen carefully to the signals your body gives that you're thirsty. When it comes, drink a glass of water. Notice any changes in body functions and energy level. Write it down.

- Often when we're tired what we really are is *dehydrated*. Next time you get tired during the day, drink a glass of water. Make note of what happens.

- For a few days replace some fluid with pure water. That's living water by the way, not dead water from a bottle – which is bad for the environment and bad for us. If you like what happens and you don't already have one, consider spending the $20 and get a filter so you can drink pure, healthy water. Enjoy.

Terra Mar

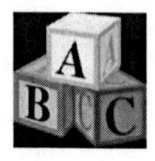

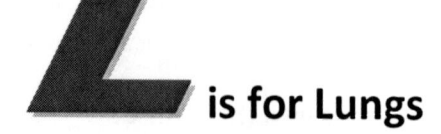

L is for Lungs

"There's so much pollution in the air now that if it weren't for our lungs there'd be no place to put it all."
-- **Robert Orben** (magician and comedian)

Common expressions such as 'a breath of spring or a breath of fresh air' are meant to show how much we love fresh air. Then there's 'breath of life' or the Yoga admonition 'change your breathing and you change your life.' Clearly we love to breathe and know we breathe to live.

So why don't we show it? At the societal level you could think it pretty crazy that we pollute the air we take into our bodies. At the individual level we smoke and ignore our body's warning signals.

As if there weren't enough other reasons to do so, cleaning up the air could reverse the staggering increases we've been experiencing in asthma and allergies over the last few decades.

According to the Asthma and Allergy Foundation of America (www.aafa.org) asthma affects an estimated 20 million Americans, and it wasn't always so.

Since the early '80s the number of asthma sufferers has been on the increase across every age, sex and racial group.

ABC's of Natural Healing

Asthma accounts for one-quarter of all emergency room visits in the U.S. each year -- 2 million.

It also accounts for more than 10 million outpatient visits and 500,000 hospitalizations

Asthma is the most common chronic condition among children. It accounts for more lost school days than any other single reason.

One of my children is among those statistics; he's part of the 50% of asthma cases that are considered allergic asthma. Watching my young son having an asthma attack ranks really high on my list of things I never wanted to experience. It was literally like watching someone trying to breathe through a straw. A small straw. It made me wish I had a magic wand.

What I lacked in magic wands, I was determined to make up for in a healthy remedy as soon as I started my **OnePlanet Herbs** business. I wanted to help not only my son and other asthma sufferers, but their loved ones who suffer right along with them.

None of the following is intended to replace proper medical care, and is for information purposes only. Given that, I felt my investment of time and research paid off. I found a powerful herb for asthma symptoms and combined it with other wonderful upper respiratory healing herbs. One of my first customers was a handsome athletic young man in his early twenties. He told me he had chronic asthma and bought the new remedy. Even I was impressed when he told me a month later that he was able to cut back his inhaler use by half.

The magic ingredient was **amor seco** *(Desmodium adscendens)*. Like most healing plants it has many uses as well as many names. Due to its powerful anti-inflammatory, anti-spasmodic and relaxant actions, it is called 'strong back' in Belize and is used for back pain. Naturopath and herbalist Rosita Arvigo wrote of strong back in her book about herbs in Belize *"Rainforest Remedies."*

She noted that in Belize the whole plant, which grows in pastures, yards and along roadsides is soaked in rum for a full day and then used for relief from back problems and muscle spasms. It is also used to treat headaches, muscle pain and joint aches, among other complaints.

Its use for asthma was first researched in Ghana, where it is also indigenous. The results were convincing enough that other studies followed.

In allergic asthma like my son has, something triggers the attack. This can be an allergen like dust or mold or an irritant like smoke or air pollution. That causes the build-up and release of histamines in the body, which result in the allergic irritation and inflammation.

The muscles around the airways tighten and spasm, the inner lining swells and gets irritated. Not only is air flow restricted, but a lot of mucus builds up as well, making it even harder to breath.

The muscle relaxation that makes amor seco valuable for back pain in Belize does the same in the upper respiratory system. In fact it does double duty – it not only helps dilate the bronchia and relax the muscles, it also helps prevent the buildup of histamines.

In other words it acts to lessen the impact and treat the symptoms. Quite fascinating. (For an in-depth account of the complex chemistry and science behind this, see Dr. Taylor's description on her www.raintree.com)

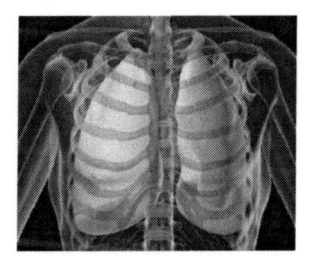

The rainforest is home to many other plants that help support the lungs. It seems indigenous healers know the value of, and seek to protect, what we too frequently take for granted: the full breath of life.

After all it is our lungs that oxygenate our blood and form are our pathway to healthy cell function throughout our bodies. They're worth a little extra care.

The eyes may be the doorway to the soul, but the lungs are the doorway to a healthy body.

Terra Mar

Lovin' up your lungtivities:

- **Enjoy lung-healthy food!** Eat antioxidant-rich food to nourish your lungs. Cruciferous veggies like broccoli, brussels sprouts, cauliflower, and kale, mustard greens cabbage and others help keep lung cells healthy. Fruit is great for lungs, especially apples. Studies indicate an apple a day can give better lung functionality. Other lung-healthy foods include yams, squash, figs, almonds and citrus fruits.

- **Smile** to your lungs and thank them.

- **Respect cigarettes** as you would any deadly enemy.

- **Exercise.** Your lungs will love you for it. So will your whole body. When you nourish your lungs you nourish all your cells.

- **Do you play the sax?** Perhaps not, but if for even 10 or 15 minutes a day you practice any wind instrument, including a recorder, it will expand your lung capacity.

- **Use visualization.** Do your own or try this one: Once you are deeply relaxed, focus on the breath. Even, deep breaths in and out. Now imagine your lungs healthy, pink, working at optimal capacity. **Breathe in.** Nice deep breath.

As you breathe in now imagine the lungs expanding bigger and bigger pushing oxygen into the bloodstream creating healthy, oxygen-rich blood.

Breathe out. Imagine your healthy red blood cells carrying the CO2 you don't need into the lungs and emptying it into the air you exhale.

Know and imagine with every deep, conscious in-breath that you enhance all the functions of your body.

With every out-breath you rid your body of what it no longer needs. Deep, conscious breathing, bringing in health, taking out what you no longer need. Every cell nourished, every cell performing at peak capacity.

Wonderful lungs. Wonderful body. Thank you lungs. Thank you body.

Come back when you're ready.

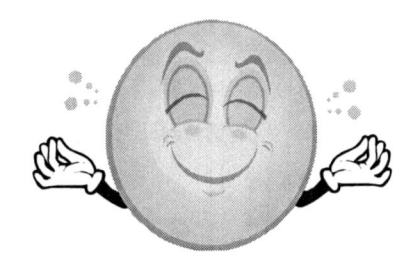

Terra Mar

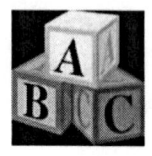

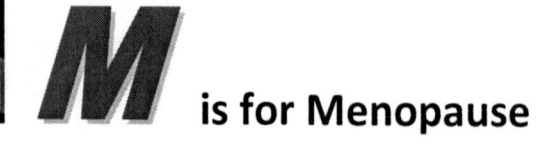

M is for Menopause

"It's okay to talk about birth, okay - then menstruation. I first started my advocacy for women's health in the field of reproductive freedom, and the next stage will be bringing menopause out of the closet."
-- Cybill Shepherd

My mother died the summer of my twelfth year, just after I got my period for the first time. When one of my aunts stated the obvious, that I was so young to lose a parent, I said: "At least my mother lived long enough to know I started my period."

I really had no idea what I was saying or why that popped out. In fact I was so uninformed about menstruation that a month later my father took the extraordinary step of calling the family doctor to our house to examine me because of my horrible intestinal pains. The doctor suddenly stopped checking my belly and asked "Do you have your period?" I nodded. He packed up and left.

If I had a daughter I would have thrown her a rite of passage party when she started menstruating. I would have searched for some wise words of parental wisdom. I would have given her a flower or a book. Something.

I know she would not have thought she was dying of a dreaded disease when the blood began to flow. (My sister straightened me out. That was my mother, not me.)

I had just entered a world I couldn't possibly grasp with no support and a mother on death's doorstep.

My comment to my aunt must have bubbled up from some primal part of me that understood what my conscious mind couldn't begin to grasp. The start of menstruation is an amazing, wonderful, awe-inspiring passage that calls out for celebration and sisterhood.

OK then, so what about the other side? What about menopause? Isn't that a passage too? You betchya! Shouldn't it too be heralded? Oh, absolutely. Fine. When? Any woman who's been there will understand. Menopause ain't over till it's over and you don't know when that's going to be.

When you start your period there aren't too many options about the way it begins. But when the cycles stop there are as many variations as women. It can happen anywhere from late 30's to early 50's or on an operating table in a flash. It can stop for months and then take you fully by surprise.

I suppose one way of honoring The Change would be to share surprise stories with other peri- or post-menopausal women. What was your most shocking and humiliating moment? Hmm...maybe not.

Terra Mar

Oh well, since I started I'll tell you mine. I trained for many years in a martial art, and one summer members of my school travelled to Sweden to a remote and beautiful island where we trained outside for several days. We all took good care of our 'gi,' our spotless white pants and jackets. Some of the jackets, especially if you use them for judo are quite long. Mine was short.

I had no reason to expect my period, but in the middle of class there it was. Bright. Shiny. RED! I had nowhere to go and no clue what to do. With no obvious alternative I gave in, figuring that if I had the discipline to continue kicking my fellow students might have the discipline (and mercy) not to stare. It worked, and I survived. During the break a tall sister-in-need with a long jacket kindly switched with me.

I can laugh now, but the unpredictability of menopause's onset is only one of its many challenging aspects. Most times you can't pinpoint when you're really, really through menopause until about a year after you stop having periods. That makes it hard to celebrate.

Besides, it's hard to want to be the center of the party when at any moment you're likely to turn red in the face and break out in a sweat.

Then there's the mood swings, the sleeplessness and a laundry list of symptoms as our bodies try desperately to recreate what they have viewed as normal for the past, oh, say 30 to 40 years.

How to get ready for the party?

Pharmaceutical Hormone Replacement Therapy (HRT) has been discredited enough that most women now think very seriously before trying it. That said and for information purposes only, if you have access to a naturopath there is the possibility of HRT using natural progesterone and Tri-est. This is not from horse urine and actually mimics the three forms of estrogen the body produces.

There are also herbal non-hormonal supports. Because there are many processes at work in menopause and so many varied symptoms, it is generally good to mix herbs for maximum benefit.

Unlike many conditions herbs are used for, menopause is not an illness – even though it can feel that way. It's a natural, if lengthy, rebalancing and an herbal therapy is used to support those processes.

Going alphabetically, let's start with **abuta** (*Cissampelos pareira*) In S. America this herb is so broadly associated as a support for women's issues that it is also known as "Midwife's Herb." A plant used for so many female hormonal balancing issues has not yet been well-researched by western science. Why am I not shocked?

Maca – again. Its properties have been referred to before in **A for Aphrodisiac, D for Disease** and in **I** as an immune enhancer. It is considered helpful for menopausal symptoms because of its documented abilities as a tonic, aphrodisiac and fertility-enhancer. Maca is a great support, but it's not a panacea.

Suma root (*Pfaffia paniculata*), also known as Brazilian ginseng is a tonic with so many wonderful qualities it's also called "for all things" throughout S. America. Not surprisingly it falls into that special category of herbal adaptogens, discussed in **F for Fatigue** and **I for Immune**.

To give you just a taste of this herb's value, in her Raintree plant database Dr. Taylor notes: "Nutritionally, suma root contains 19 different amino acids, a large number of electrolytes, trace minerals, iron, magnesium, zinc, vitamins A, B1, B2, E, K, and pantothenic acid."

There are others as well. I've already mentioned both **chuchuhuasi** and **sarsaparilla in F is for Fatigue**. Both help balance hormones. Then there's **damiana, mulungu** and **passionflower**, which counter anxiety and support relaxation and restful sleep.

The list of menopausal symptoms is long; the list of supporting herbs from the Amazon rainforest may be even longer.

A word about the guys

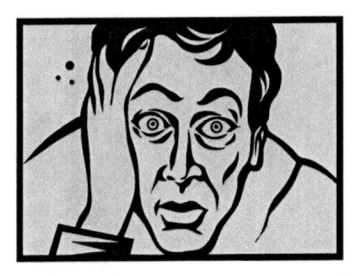

Men of a certain age: if you think it's only your woman who's moody, grumpy, not sleeping well and less interested in sex you're probably not looking much in your internal mirror. Apparently the reduced testosterone levels in men also brings about surprisingly similar symptoms to what women experience, including thinning bones, hot flashes, sweats, and increased body fat.

Don't get angry at me. I'm just repeating what the docs are finding. Current discussion is underway as to whether to spring male menopause from the isolated world of women's jokes and move it into the light of a medical condition -- not illness guys, just another rite of passage. They even have a separate name – andropause, referring to the lowered testosterone level.

Whether you're male or female, you may never experience strong symptoms. If so, be grateful. For the rest of us, consider the options, talk to health care professionals, and consider how you can improve your situation.

Terra Mar

Meanwhile, some parting thoughts:

- CELEBRATE, and make it a bash to remember!

- If you are pre-menopausal, menopausal, or newly post-menopausal, document your fluctuations and have a fluctuation party! You could give prizes for the most fluctuations or most symptoms, or...

- Throw a *this is my last period... or not*, party.

- Have a hot flash party.

- Dress up. Dance. Laugh about it. Bring it out of the closet and into the streets!

- Invite younger and older women to a *change of life is cool* party. Let the younger women know before it's upon them that they too can pick a time to celebrate their change. Have the older women share their stories.

- Whatever you choose, remember to include some elders, women who are definitely post-menopausal and found new excitement, energy, and creativity in that freedom.

N is for Nature

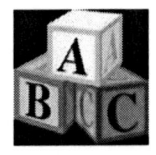

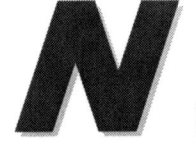

"We first knew you a feeble plant which wanted a little earth whereon to grow. We gave it to you; and afterward, when we could have trod you under our feet, we watered and protected you; and now you have grown to be a mighty tree, whose top reaches the clouds, and whose branches overspread the whole land, whilst we, who were the tall pines of the forest, have become a feeble plant and need your protection." -- **Sogoyewapha**, (Red Jacket), Seneca Nation

I don't want to say I told you so, but, well. I did. I told you how important Nature is. Mostly I have been pointing out that Nature is part of what we are, and that we need our connection to it not only to save the planet but our souls as well.

Now an article I found in the Boston Globe points out just how important Nature is to our *brain*. I'd like to take the opportunity of **N** not to gloat (further), but to offer some recommendations for the city dwellers among us.

The good news is that with relatively small adjustments we can help our all-important brain cells. I had planned to do **N** for neuroprotective and highlight the herb **samambaia**, which is brilliant for the brain. This is really not so far off; simply another approach to being neurowise.

Take me to the village...please

As you probably know, we humans are hard-wired for village life. We are communal by nature. Small groups, a sense of community, knowing our neighbors, familiarity with our neighborhoods, these are all natural for us. If it sounds like an idyllic life from long ago, you got that part right as well. That's where it is for most of us – in the past. In fact for the first time in human history over half the population of the world lives in cities.

City life may conjure up fun images like bars, theater, opera, coffee houses, good restaurants, art walks and pretty much whatever tickles your fancy. For the upper one percent of the world's population that's at our beck and call. But science has shown what most of us in the 99 percent already knew – the city can be an unnatural, overwhelming, alienating energy drain. Which doesn't mean it can't also be cool and hip and fun. But hard on us it is.

In a study at the University of Michigan, a monitored group walked in an arboretum while another did the same in downtown. The city strollers returned in a worse mood and scored significantly lower on *attention and working memory* tests. Additionally, pictures of city scenes led to "measurable impairments," while pictures of nature correlated with higher scores on attention and memory-based tests.

Buddhism says enlightenment is like our eyelashes; too close for us to notice. Perhaps peace of mind and improved performance are as simple as a walk in the park.

I lived in Europe, mostly in Vienna, for many years and returned to the States with my two children when they were in their early teens. We moved to the Seattle area thinking that for two kids raised in Europe the slower pace of the west coast would be an easier transition. Boy had I forgotten what the U.S. was like!

The billboards, the lights, advertisements everywhere, huge stores with vast amounts of merchandise, and all of that while having to navigate a new town... There were days, actually many of them, where one of the kids would ask if we could just go home and rest. All three of us were exhausted from the input. And we were coming from a big city!

Our other safe haven was a small, relatively unpopulated beach on Puget Sound. We spent time there whenever we could. We were like HSPs in an overcrowded room with flashing lights.

The theory of Highly Sensitive People (HSP) is neither positive nor negative; it refers to input sensitivity and how quickly a person gets overloaded and goes into overwhelm. HSPs' brains are a little on overload all the time, so additional input from crowds, lights, and other stimuli tends to send HSPs over the edge. The major recommendations to soothe HSPs are quiet time and time in nature. *To a greater or lesser degree, the city turns us all into HSPs.*

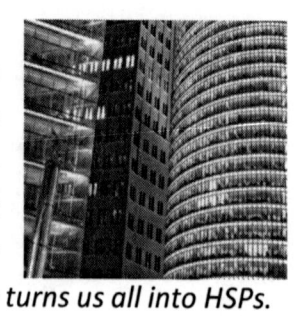

I can't resist quoting from the article about the city because the conclusions are so simple, and in a sane world would not need scientific validation. But our world is nothing if not crazy, so here we go:

"One of the main forces at work is a stark lack of nature, which is surprisingly beneficial for the brain. Studies have demonstrated, that hospital patients recover more quickly when they can see trees from their windows, and that women living in public housing are better able to focus when their apartment overlooks a grassy courtyard.

Even these fleeting glimpses of nature improve brain performance, it seems, because they provide a mental break from the urban roil."

Simply by navigating urban density as we are assaulted by noise, crowds, bright lights big city, our poor prefrontal cortex's functionality gets zapped. This is not a good thing. It means our brains get hit with a double whammy because that little piece of brain has two important functions. It helps us focus and helps us maintain control.

When it's overloaded we are less able to focus our attention and hold things in memory. At the same time self-control and good judgment are asleep at the wheel. So here we are surrounded by temptations and distractions and our natural ability to focus and resist them is short-circuited by the very distractions that call to us.

We may end up buying things we don't need, get taken in by city slickers, or simply frazzled without knowing why. It's certainly no wonder that quick fixes, fast food, and play money at ATM's are established pieces of our urban landscapes.

The city is dead. Long live the city!

Oddly enough, even the bad parts ain't all bad. No need to give up our day jobs and apartments or craft an epitaph on the city. Like democracy or baking bread it's messy, but it works. Obviously not all our brain cells get destroyed because the city is a hub of cultural and intellectual activity, scientific breakthroughs and entrepreneurial spirit,

Apparently it is exactly the alienation, confusion, and complexity of urban life that challenge the human spirit and intellect. Our creative and innovative spirit is encouraged by the lack of predictability, by coping with the unanticipated, the chance meeting with strangers

Terra Mar

who think and act in unexpected ways, and the difficulties of survival in the urban jungle.

What happens to you in the city? That question still needs to be answered. Everything else is statistics, and as such irrelevant to the life experience of a single individual. What happens to you after a day in the 'real' world? When you come back home are you ready to pick up a paintbrush, take a class, read a book or write one? Or are you ready to kick the dog, yell at the kids, vegg out on the sofa and collapse into bed?

Be honest, because there is no right or wrong answer. It's only information, data without judgment. Once you know what city life does to *your* inner life, you can decide how to proceed.

Nature is. Each of us decides when, how, or whether we want to partner with her.

As the quote pointed out, the good news is that a little nature goes a long way. While scientists and urban planners explore ways to improve cities by adding more trees, more parks, more plants and more variety of plants, (duh) we don't have to wait for the experts. We can improve our thinking, brain function, decision-making capacity, energy level, and overall health with a few simple steps.

Naturcizes:

- Even if we live in the densest of urban jungles, even if we live in a tiny apartment, we can still get ourselves something living – house plants or flowers from the market. We can get an easy-care animal like a turtle or a fish, or both.

- Remember the days of the terrarium? A little ecosystem in a glass container. We could build our own terrarium with compatible plants.

- We can designate an area of our home as a nature preserve and fill it with plants and herbs. A plant light helps to focus attention on it.

- Take a few minutes in the morning to appreciate your natural area. Thank your life forms, plant or animal, and tell them you'll think of them during the day.

- Think of them during the day. When you feel yourself stressed, tired or overwhelmed imagine and remember your morning interaction with the nature you brought into your life. Breathe in the memories and breathe out the stress.

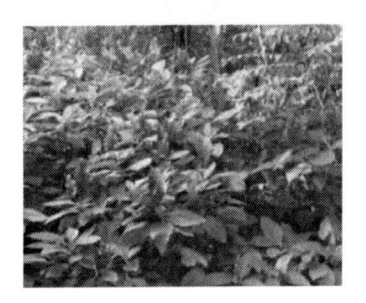

Terra Mar

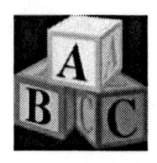

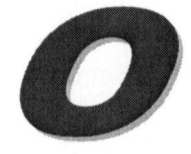

O is for Obesity

"To say that obesity is caused by merely consuming too many calories is like saying that the only cause of the American Revolution was the Boston Tea Party."
-- **Adelle Davis** (pioneer in nutrition, author of "Let's Eat Right to Keepse Fit," hated by the corporate food industry she outspokenly attacked)

When I went to Rio I was introduced to porangaba. I drank it several times as a tea, and saw it at the beach in drinks as well. It turned out to be **chá de bugre** *(Cordia salicifolia)* under another name, currently hitting the U.S. market as an herbal weight loss product.

It's really popular there, although the women I met in Rio didn't look like they needed any weight loss. Maybe it's something in the drinking water, or that they don't seem to sleep much. Or the chá de bugre

I certainly had no illusions that I'd look like the Brazilian women, but kept drinking chá de bugre on a regular basis for a while after I got back to the States. My reaction was textbook. It's not supposed to kill your appetite, just give you a feeling of satisfaction with less food.

The first few days I didn't notice a difference, but after about three days I remember thinking I'm eating less. I noticed I was leaving food on my plate that I would normally have eaten and began wondering why my stomach seemed to have shrunk. Then I made the connection.

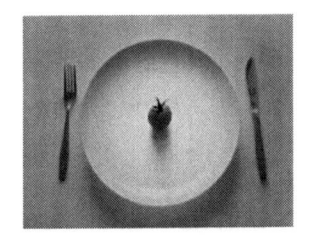

You could say memories of Rio or placebo effect, but I did take off weight. Meanwhile I had learned that chá de bugre was also reputed to break up cellulite and act as a heart tonic as well. A winning combination indeed. So...

Is chá de bugre the silver bullet we've all been waiting for?

How to put this gently. NO! NO! and HELL NO! Does it do what it says it will? I'm convinced it does. *But that doesn't mean that you or I will.* At the end of the day, that's the point. I believe most of us know what's healthy to eat and how much of it is good for us. I also believe that temptation, life style, and emotions are powerful contributors to our eating obsessions.

Food, for many of us, is our drug of choice.

Remember the guy who lost like a million pounds by eating at Subway every day? Assuming that actually happened, and assuming he kept the weight off, my conclusion is that when it comes to taking off weight, anything can work. The corollary is that it is equally likely that nothing will work.

Terra Mar

It's not about a silver bullet somewhere out there. It's not about a particular diet, a new fad, or a fabulous herb. I do believe there is a silver bullet, a magic ingredient, and a real showstopper.

I believe, for better or worse, it's you and your own self-image.

Speaking for myself, I know exactly the weight at which I stopped losing, and I know exactly how connected it is to my own self-image.

I've taught enough weight control classes to know three things:

1. *Habits prevail.* They are far stronger than any food, fad or diet.

2. *Will power is short-lived.* It can get you started, but it won't last.

3. *Food is not the issue.* It's the symptom.

I also know this:

We can change our eating habits permanently.

We can change our relationship to food permanently.

We can keep weight off permanently.

To do so requires enthusiastic cooperation from the strongest part of our self – our subconscious mind. Our self-image resides there, and from it we create an outer reflection of our inner image. Often that's the bad news, but it's also the good news.

The other piece of good news is that we continue to create our self-image every night when we go to sleep and every morning when we wake up. That means if we don't like it we **can** change it.

Once our subconscious mind is excited and fully on board about a different self-image it will work as hard to reflect that as it did the old one. That's when change happens. Suddenly it's not a diet, it's just a better way of eating, exercise is finally fun, not a chore. What once had been a struggle, now is a piece of cake, if you'll pardon the expression.

There are techniques for making those powerful self-image changes. If you're interested in pursuing it I'd suggest some good hypnotherapy tapes or a visit to a well-trained hypnotherapist. It's not the only method, but it's a powerful and effective one.

So far I've been talking about personal responsibility. I believe in that and I know you do if you're reading a book about health and herbs. We agree that as grown-ups we are responsible for what we put in our mouths, and I don't want to put a qualifier on that. Buuut… I have to.

Because obesity is not just an individual problem. It's way past that. It's beyond young women wanting to fit into a size 2, or trying to look like a movie star. It's

Terra Mar

beyond mature women worrying about an extra five pounds. Way. In fact this is way past anything we've ever known in human history.

It's not just you. Not by a long shot

As you may remember from **N**, when we separate from Nature, we become vulnerable to the temptations that surround us. If we combine the advertising dollars spent by the multi-billion dollar food industry with the fact that more people than ever before live in the city we begin to get a sense of what is foisted upon us daily.

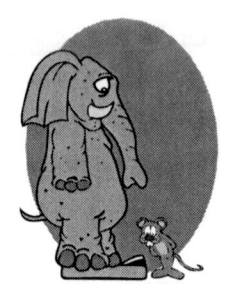

If you've read books like *"Fast Food Nation"* or *"The Omnivore's Dilemma"* you get a sense of what it means to have a handful of corporations controlling around 80 percent of our food options.

We could add that the earth in which we grow our food has fewer nutrients than at any time in history. Throw into the mix that we live in a whirlwind of stress, speed, and constant demands on our time and energy. We could easily add in a dozen other stressors, but it's not necessary.

The picture of what we're up against is clear and indisputable. Sadly statistics abound to prove it. In an intergenerational mirror, it is powerfully reflected back to us in the staggering increases of diseases in our children – obesity, diabetes, ADHD, allergies, and asthma.

How do we cope when it feels so big?

The answer is a bit paradoxical. Sometimes it's easier to cope with something really huge than our daily mini-dramas. It's all about motivation. When I was diagnosed with stage 3 breast cancer, trust me, it felt Big. But so did my desire to live and regain my health. It was even bigger than I realized at the time.

It was so deep and powerful a part of me that I had no problem making the necessary changes and taking the necessary medical steps. As overwhelming, abhorrent, or frightening as they may have seemed to a healthy person, to me it was simply another step in my journey to wellness.

I used Eastern, Earth-based and Western medicine to their fullest. *It was natural and instinctive – and I didn't even realize it.* My deepest survival instincts had kicked in and my subconscious mind had taken over. The same miracles can happen with your relationship with food. It can be that easy and natural.

I'm going to suggest a sure-fire way to get started. This may not be the moment or the issue for you and that's fine. It will be here if you ever need it. Otherwise, enjoy, and send your judgmental self to the movies before, during and after you do this!!

Terra Mar

Daring Changercise:

- Finding the subconscious. To me, this is the first step to any BIG change. We have to go in there and get the attention of our own subconscious mind. As I said before, there are good CD's for this, but here's something you can try right now. The principle is exactly the same.

- To get to the subconscious mind we need to quiet the mental chatter and relax. That's it. The more we relax, the more quiet our conscious mind becomes. The quieter it is, the more we relax.

- The subconscious mind is like a huge container. It holds old memories, belief systems, our flight or fight reflex and protective mechanisms. It's not a thinking part of us in the way our conscious mind is. It's passive and can't tell the difference between something real and something strongly, repeatedly and emotionally imagined. Put in positive suggestions combined with powerful emotional beliefs in a very relaxed state, and out comes the desired change.

- Find a comfortable position and a time when you can turn off your cell phone and you won't be disturbed for at least 10 – 15 minutes. If life is hectic, this could be right before you sleep or before you hurl yourself out of bed in the morning. They're both ideal times because in those half waking moments the veil is quite thin between our active mind and our inner world.

Find your best way to relax. A good method is to take each body part, focus on it, and tell it to relax. Another good one is to count yourself down from 20 to 1, slowing your breathing, and using the (unspoken) word 'relax' after each number. Any technique you know that helps you relax deeply is fine.

Now explain to your subconscious mind what you want. Show it the image of the healthy body you want to have. Be enthusiastic about it, like you're trying to get a little kid excited about a new game. Be descriptive, detailed, repetitive, and as enthusiastic as a cheerleader. Take as much time for this as you want, but it needs at least a solid 5 – 10 minutes. Especially the first time.

Thank your subconscious for listening and head back out.

- Smile. You just accomplished a lot more than you may realize.

- Be prepared to repeat this. You didn't get into your current self-concept in a day. Give yourself a month of doing this daily. It gets easier and more powerful every time you do it.

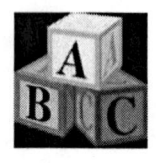

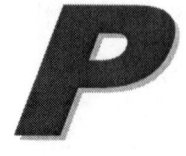

Terra Mar

P is for Pacing

"What is any art but a mould in which to imprison for a moment the shining elusive element which is life itself - life hurrying past us and running away, too strong to stop, too sweet to lose." -- **Willa S. Cather** (Pulitzer Prize winning American author, 1873-1947)

For the sake of discussion, let's say you're going to run a marathon. How will you prepare? You'll need to build your muscles, expand your lung capacity, stretch to stay limber, and you'll need to learn how to pace yourself. Pacing is a huge part of success in any long-term endeavor.

This, you may say, is neither news nor rocket science. Ahh, so you say now. But what happens when we apply the same principles to our lives?

I was keenly aware of many life style differences between life in Europe and life in the States, but I hadn't thought about the difference between Europeans and Americans until I worked a stint as a coordinator for an MBA student exchange program. It was my job to welcome the American Masters students and take them out for a day of touring.

I organized walking tours in three separate towns, each with a different Austrian flair. This also included a visit to a famous museum, a trip to a popular lake resort, and a visit to spectacular cathedral. We needed to travel in our chartered bus from one place to the other, and I was concerned it was too ambitious for one day, especially since we were going out that evening.

I had been away from the States too long. I thought the reaction of my European friends – are you crazy? -- meant I had found the right balance. Anything but! My itinerary was way too ambitious for Europeans -- not for Americans.

It turned into a cultural mismatch and a day from hell. I had to spontaneously add in an event in a fourth town, one as far from Vienna as I could get to use up additional time. Even so we arrived back earlier than planned. I was utterly exhausted. They were bored.

At the lake resort my fatal miscalculation was painfully obvious. Europeans would have walked the lake in small groups, then sat down at the tables for a coffee, and checked out the scenery. Knowing I was planning for Americans, I had crunched the timetable down to about an hour; the Americans were done in 15 minutes.

Not one person made it around the (small) lake. No groups formed. No one sat down at the tables. No one ordered anything to drink. They came back to the bus in one's and two's, candy and ice cream in hand, wanting to know what was next.

Terra Mar

Been that, done there.

Certainly many Americans would make the argument that this group had paced itself a little faster than Europeans, but so what. In my opinion, the 'what' is that they not only missed some historic, unique, spectacular sites, but more importantly they missed the feeling of being connected.

They missed out on appreciating a small and simple, seemingly unworthy lake, just as I had done years earlier. They overlooked architecture and sensory inputs in a cathedral that had witnessed spiritual and religious ecstasy. They had outpaced their connection to the world around them.

If our pace is too fast, we outpace the part of us that longs for connection to others, to Nature, to the Earth.

At least one shamanic tradition holds that the soul can travel only as fast as a horse can run. We, and our souls, need time. It's part of village life, part of what we long for when we miss a sense of community.

My martial arts teacher travelled internationally a great deal. Often on returning home he would say his soul hadn't come back yet. Generally it arrived a few days later and he felt whole again.

Attached to slower pace is the connection to place, to the moment, and to the world around us. If we set the wrong pace in a marathon we lose the race; in a lifetime we lose relationships and lasting memories.

One way to slow ourselves down enough to be present at any time, anywhere is through gratitude. If we feel gratitude for what we are experiencing we place ourselves squarely into the moment. It has been shown to improve health by changing our physiology, and it is considered one of the most powerful of all states of being.

Each of the letters in this book has a 'takeaway,' an exercise, an action, or a thought attached. Several present wonderful rainforest herbs that are new to many readers. Why do some readers take action and others not? Why will some try a new herb or approach while others don't?

Among the many possible reasons, I would suggest that we need to have enough pain and suffering with the ways we are used to before we are willing to challenge ourselves with something new. Frequently it means we have to change pace.

The ability to slow down and change pace is a valuable tool that encourages change, attentiveness, and productivity. We seek to understand and protect what we notice and connect with, whether it's a new healing modality, our neighborhood, or the rainforest.

Check and change:

The following four tips can help you check and change pacing.

🌿 Food

Almost 20 years ago a new concept emerged from a country already associated with healthy eating – Italy. The movement became known as 'Slow Food.' Today it has over 80,000 members in 100 countries. It was founded to "counteract the disappearance of local food traditions and people's dwindling interest in the food they eat, where it comes from, how it tastes and how our food choices affect the rest of the world."

The Slow Food movement (www.slowfood.org) is an open invitation to consider anew our interest in food and the many aromas and flavors of food. As well, it is an opportunity to examine the many issues surrounding food.

Food is a great way to check ourselves. Want a really, really simple way to break into that? It's easy, but challenging. Count your bites and chew each bite 50 times.

You'll be amazed at how far off you're likely to be when you start. It's considered an optimal number of bites for digestion, but it's an intense meditation.

🌸 Breath

Another simple and hugely challenging change is through the breath. If you want a challenge that makes 50 bites seem easy, focus only on your breath for two full minutes. If you notice your mind wandering, bring it back to the breath. If that's too much, start with one minute.

You don't need a mudra or lotus position. You can be anywhere, anytime. Keep it simple.

🌸 Quiet

Pretend you've been sent off for quiet time. This is time out from other people, phones, screens, music and all disturbances. How much can you take and still feel good about the quiet? Whatever your time is, gently increase it as you plateau.

It's really not a punishment. It's more a detox.

🌸 Play

Do you play? Assuming you are a grown-up, what is play for you? Take a moment and jot down the top three ways you play. Games, baths, gardening, books, Wii, a craft or other hobby...

Whatever it is build it into your week. Spend a little more time with it than usual, or add it in again if it has fallen by the wayside.

Terra Mar

> Do you have another way to check your pacing and slow it to appreciate the world around you and your connection to it even more than you do now?

I'll leave you with this old joke

An American businessman was at the pier of a coastal Mexican village when a small boat docked with one fisherman and several large yellow fin tuna. The American complimented him on the fish and asked how long it took to catch them. The man replied only a little while. The American asked why he hadn't stayed out longer to catch more, to which the man answered he had enough fish.

The American asked: "But what do you do with the rest of your time?"

"I sleep late, fish a little, play with my children, take a siesta with my wife Maria, stroll into the village where I sip wine and play guitar with my friends."

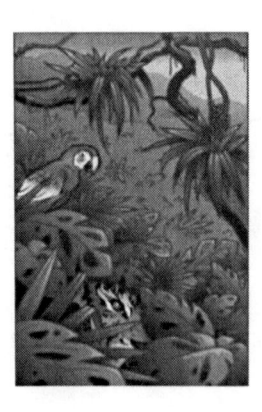

The American scoffed, "I know business, and I'll help you. First, spend more time fishing and with the proceeds, buy a bigger boat. With the money from the extra catch you can buy more boats. Eventually you will have a whole fleet.

Instead of selling to a middleman you sell directly to the processor. Finally you open your own cannery, then you control the product from catch to distribution. You will become very wealthy."

The fisherman asked, "But señor, how long will this all take?"

To which the American replied, "15-20 years."

"But what then, señor?"

The American laughed. "That's the best part. When the time is right you sell your company and walk away with millions."

"Ah, and then señor?"

The American paused for some time before replying: "Then you retire. You could move to a coastal village, fish a little, play with your grandchildren, take a siesta with your wife, stroll to the village in the evenings, sip wine and play guitar with your friends."

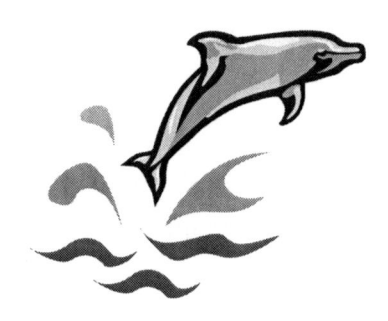

Terra Mar

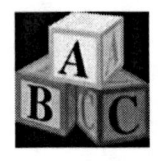

Q is for Quechua

"Andean music is is a waterfall/encountered in a quiet forest:/playful and powerful at the same time.
Andean music is the voice of the wind/that howls among the high rocks: nothing but air, but nevertheless very strong.
Andean music is the flight of the condor/making a design against the sky: it appears to be art, but gives sustenance." -- **June Ireland** translated from Quechua (http://www.andes.org/ poems.html)

I ended **P** with a joke and now I have to start **Q** with one. This is well-known in Europe.

Q. What's a person who speaks three languages?
A. Trilingual

Q. What's a person who speaks two languages?
A. Bilingual

Q. What's a person who speaks one language?
A. American

We Americans accomplish so much but tend not to learn other languages. More's the pity because hidden in other languages are unfamiliar ways of thinking, living and belief systems.

By those who speak it, Quechua it is called Runasimi, meaning 'mouth of the people.' It was the language of the Inca Empire of Peru. Although the takeover by Conquistadores decimated the population, survivors spread to many places in S. America, and the language endured, sort of.

What is collectively known as Quechua is a vastly divergent dialect chain that covers most indigenous people in the west of South America. The Quechua-speaking people migrated widely, both south along the Andes and east into the rainforest of the Amazon Basin. This early divergence in their migration paths created distinct mountain- and jungle- Quechua identities and cultures.

Estimates of the number of people speaking Quechua vary enormously, mostly depending on whether all dialects are included. No matter how you add it up though, it is the most widely-spoken indigenous language in the Americas.

Even though the dialects are so diverse that a speaker in Bolivia may not understand the Quechua of Peru, Argentina, Ecuador or Brazil, the best estimate is that there exist somewhere between seven and ten million speakers of the language.

Why am I devoting a letter chapter to Quechua? Because Q is hard? Neh. I had a bunch of other ideas to choose from. I picked it because the survival of a language and the survival of a culture are inextricable. And our world can't afford more of this loss.

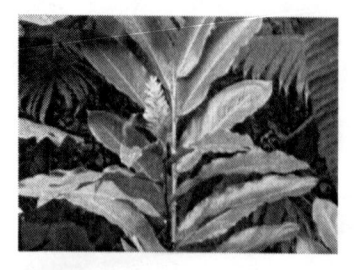

The phenomenon of rainforest destruction and the simultaneous extinction of indigenous tribes is a prime example. At our own peril, we watch as the land gets decimated, the cultural fabric of rainforest peoples unravels, and the youth assimilate or disappear.

One of the indicators of the disappearing rainforest cultures is the loss of shamans. Whatever your spiritual or religious beliefs, they probably do not center around shamanism. Not so in earth-based cultures.

Shamanism is an iconic part of the heritage of all indigenous cultures. For rainforest peoples, they are not only an essential part of daily life, ceremony and survival, but also the carriers of healing plant knowledge from generation to generation. This worked quite well throughout human history until we non-rainforest dwellers came on the scene.

The 200,000 square miles of the Amazon lost to short-sighted commercial interests in the last few decades have changed the balance forever. Along with a quickening of this destructive pattern, the old shamans are dying off without a cadre of new ones to take their place. If they survive the encroachment, their cultures are upended. As young people assimilate, they lose interest in the old ways.

I've been trying to think of an equivalent for us and haven't been able to come up with an answer. Except for one disturbing image that keeps coming into my mind. I'd say it's unthinkable, except that I'm thinking it. Here goes:

What would it be like if most young women decided they did not want to be mothers and instead put their newborns into orphanages? I know it sounds like a sci-fi plot, but I can't come any closer. Mothers are both symbol and soul of our society. If we lost that with no young girls to take their place our foundations would crumble.

In the case of rainforest shamans, their dwindling numbers represents an incalculable loss to their own society and it is also devastating to us and our future. People used to think that shamans' plant knowledge was gained thousands of years ago and somewhat statically handed down in the oral tradition. A recent study shows the learning is ongoing.

When ethnobotanists studied medicinal plant use by recently contacted tribes, they found plants for treating fungal infections, insect and snake bites, dental ailments, parasites, pains and traumatic injuries.

What they did not find were treatments for western diseases. However, tribes that had a history of ongoing contact with the outside world had hundreds of medicinal plants to counteract the new western diseases facing the people.

No one knows how the shamans gained this knowledge. Westerners wonder, forest dwellers say the spirits of the rainforest taught them. The fact remains that disappearing shamans take with them information so vital that we are losing the only crucial link between the pharmacopeia of healing that is the rainforest and the potential eradication of diseases such as cancer, AIDS, heart disease, diabetes, asthma, and the common cold.

Dr. Mark Plotkin, an ethnobotanist who spent decades in the Amazon noted that:

"*Every time a shaman dies, it is as if a library burned down.*"

Consumers spend about $6 billion a year on tropically-derived pharmaceuticals. Will we figure out what we're destroying before we lose it all?

Every day we lose plant species forever. I believe there's enough scientific validation for us to now say *answers to life-saving cures are in the rainforests.*

To find them will require awareness and active support at all levels — from government, business, non-government organizations, and consumers. It will require the political will to carry out research that is equitable to rainforest inhabitants, that preserves the integrity of land and culture and that is not biased by wealthy companies seeking to patent a tiny piece of a larger living mosaic, but is motivated enough to support generic research.

While I'm dreaming, I'd like to add that we will also need more devoted folks who understand the value of learning the language of people we want to work with. Language shapes thinking, thinking shapes people, and people shape cultures.

In the case of Quechua, that means learning far more words than condor and llama. It means opening to a different, vastly older, and more spirit-oriented world view than our own.

Language rethink

There's an old adage about being very careful what you set your heart on because you'll surely achieve it. In a similar vein I believe we need to be careful with our language because it helps form us, limit or expand us, and impacts the world around us, sometimes indelibly.

Language offers us an opportunity to be more conscious. One way to do that is to look with a fresh eye at old words.

If you've learned a second language you've probably laughed about some of the idioms. That's because, un-

Terra Mar

like the native speaker, you hear them literally. I could give pages of examples of this, but I'll give two. Perhaps you have your own.

In Austria when I was first learning German I was sitting with two native speakers, my roommate and her friend. Apparently my roommate had said something nice to him, which I didn't get. I did understand a simpler phrase though. He said "Thank you for the flowers."

I thought it was sweet that she had given him flowers, but I didn't see any. I finally leaned over and asked her in English where the flowers were. She translated and they both had kicks and giggles for the week. 'Danke fuer die Blumen' was simply a polite way of saying 'thank you' for a compliment.

Another time my Austrian friends were poking fun at the antics of someone who was pretty wild. They thought he was crazy and said he had a "bird in the head." I was the only one who found that a hilarious image, a bird flying around in a person's head.

Years later, when I was back in the States someone said 'bats in the belfry;' same meaning, but I never found it funny. The tables had turned (there's another one).

Languacizes:

- Exploring language can help us expand our thinking and sensitize us cross-culturally. Do you have a favorite phrase or idiom? Listen to yourself from the point of view of someone who hears you literally. Here's a simple one: "He's driving me crazy." One might wonder why you would think that when you're not in a car.

- If you want to take this a step further, it might be fun to consider what concepts we have a lot of words to express — like dirt or cold. Language is living and impacts us at all levels. What do you come up with? What are the nuances, similarities or differences in the synonyms? What does it say about our culture?

- Do our idioms express the values and thinking we want others to associate with us?

"Puma and moon
constellation of Llama, wind and ice
Beautiful enchantment.
Night in the highlands;
thus am I fed."
-- **June Ireland** from: 'The Puma Comes By Night'

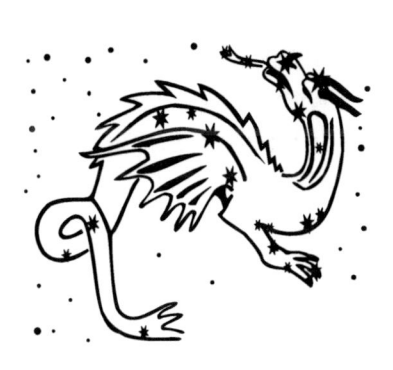

Terra Mar

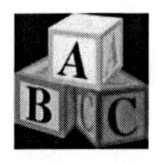

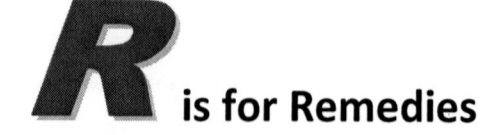

R is for Remedies

"Good for the body is the work of the body, good for the soul the work of the soul, and good for either the work of the other." -- **Henry David Thoreau**

I have talked about herbs and herbal remedies and made lots of suggestions about which herbs are good for what ailments. I think it's time to step back and see what is behind an herbal remedy. A remedy from China may be quite different from a rainforest mix or one from India or the U.S. But how, and why?

Compared to other huge topics, this one is bigger than huge. It's gigantic. It includes what a plant is, how plants impact humans, how human body systems work, and global differences in history, geography, culture and belief systems. All of these infuse what will be in an herbal remedy.

Another reason this topic is huge is because herbal healing is old. I mean really, really old. As old as (human) time, and that's a lot of history. Perhaps you remember the herb drawings found in a cave that dated back into the mists of who knows when. Maybe 20,000 years ago. Or the herbs found from 80,000 years ago.

There are indicators showing an unbroken chain of use over millennia. In China, and in Mesopotamia under the Sumerians recorded herbal use dates back some 5,000 years. That's 3,000 years Before Christ (BC)! In India, Ayurvedic medicinal herbs have been recorded in the Vedas, or ancient holy books.

The Rig Veda includes over 60 medicinal preparations. The Rig Veda was written over 6,000 years ago.

There are four major divisions in approaching herbal remedies. The differences break down along nothing less than a society's world view.

Chinese herbal medicine

All Chinese herbal therapies are based on the balance of opposites, yin and yang, and on increasing the free flow of energy (qi) throughout the body's energy channels.

No symptom or body system is treated in isolation, nor from a western perspective, even treated directly. From the Chinese herbal medicine perspective this makes sense because the herbalist is seeking out and treating not the immediate symptom, but the underlying imbalance.

This unique world view infuses all aspects of Chinese healing and has created a long and unbroken tradition of herbal healing with many offshoots. They all share the belief that health involves free energy flow and a balance of yin and yang. Acupuncture, tai chi, qigong, dietary approaches, and other natural treatments all combine energy flow and balancing of opposites.

As discussed in **H is for Herbs**, the word 'herb' is used loosely when applied to herbal medicine. In Chinese herbalism the term is loose enough to be almost unrecognizable to westerners. It includes shells, animal body parts and kelp as well as unfamiliar roots, tubers, leaves, shoots, seeds, bushes and flowers.

Ayurvedic medicine

Even the word ayurveda is old. It is derived from two Sanskrit words – Ayu meaning life, and Veda, meaning knowledge or science.

Like Chinese herbal medicine, ayurvedic treatment emphasizes mind, body, and spirit as interconnected when assessing disease and approaching prevention and treatment. Another similarity is the existence of many offshoots into interrelated modalities including yoga, breath work, various forms of cleansing and lifestyle and dietary recommendations.

Unlike Chinese herbalism, many of the most commonly prescribed ayurvedic herbs are not highly esoteric. You may not know ashwaganda or boswellia, although both are gaining a great deal of recognition in the west. But you're very likely to know turmeric, ginger, or myrrh.

Chinese medicine practitioners seek balance in body, mind, spirit by balancing the two opposites of yin and yang. Ayurveda practitioners do the same by balancing three elemental dynamics. Each person is considered a blend of three 'doshas,' or vital energies- vata, pitta and kapha.

By the time we are adults, all of us are out of balance to some degree. Ayurveda seeks to restore that essential harmony.

Because of the importance both these old traditions place on energetic balance, it is a natural outcome that they place a large emphasis on *prevention* of disease. By seeking to balance underlying disharmonies, both treat the *patient* rather than the disease.

For those of us used to western allopathic medical treatments, this is quite a stretch. In ancient China doctors were paid only when their patients stayed healthy or were healed from an illness. On the ladder of respectability, the most revered doctor was the one whose patients never got ill.

How would that work if we applied it to managed care? Sigh.

Indigenous herbalism

Indigenous herbal use among native populations around the world also dates back thousands of years. Herbal remedies from rainforest dwellers have been a part of life, culture, healing, and ceremony since prehistoric times.

As long as there have been witch doctors and shamans there has been herbal healing.

Western herbalism was once part of this tradition, but then the druids and healers/witches of Europe were hunted down and the old ways went into hiding.

When herbalism reemerged in Europe it was along with the Enlightenment and the rise of science. In the east however, herbal traditions remained unbroken for over 5,000 years.

Indigenous herbal healing has an especially strong focus on plant spirits. Plant spirits guide healers, teach them, and support them in their work. Most rainforest and other earth-based cultures are anthropomorphic; believing all of Nature is alive. The spirits of Nature and especially those of plants, still infuse the work of today's shamanic healers.

Which leads us to the new kid on the block

Relatively speaking, the western herbalism we know today is a baby, though its deepest roots lie in the western herbalism of antiquity.

Comparing it with modern allopathic medicine, the latter is fully reactive, combating disease when and where it occurs. Allopathic medicine views systems and organs in isolation, and seeks to understand a single cause of a single condition and find a targeted cure.

Western herbalism is gaining new recognition as a means of providing more of a focus on support for the whole person. Known in this context as complementary medicine, herbal remedies along with acupuncture, massage and a wide array of holistic methods are used to augment the reach of modern western medicine.

All herbal remedies

Herbalists view the interactions among healer, healing, and patient as a web of relationships and *all* herbal remedies stem from that view. All herbal traditions also believe in the synergy and wider reach of plants working in combination. This is why most herbal remedies include several herbs.

They have a wider reach and are more broadly able to effect healing. Herbal remedies are designed to activate our own healing energies, strengthen our ability to cope with attacks from without and imbalances from within.

Not to diss pharmaceuticals, because as I've said repeatedly they have their place. But herbal remedies tend to be reasonably priced, have vastly fewer side-effects than pharmaceuticals, seek to normalize our entire physiology, and soothe our spirit.

Herbs to play with

🌿 In **H is for Herbs** you got to make a bath infusion. Now you can try your hand at making your own remedy to ingest. Here is an easy place to start....

But first, while I advocate for responsible herb use, it is also important to trust your own ability to put together simple remedies. We all have ongoing relationships with herbs, even if only for cooking.

Mint, sage and other common culinary herbs do just fine in the bath or as tea. Lavender, chamomile, orange peel and lemon peel are household items and can also be used in simple remedies for the bath and in teas.

🌿 You don't need to be a trained herbalist to play with, savor, and benefit from herbs

Are there any herbs you are familiar with and wouldn't want to be without? How about putting them into a bath sachet or a simple tea?

Here's a suggestion for a relaxing, tasty herbal tea remedy. Take it any time you want to feel relaxed and soothed. It's great for evening, as the passionflower will definitely provide a deep feeling of relaxation.

You'll notice these are not all rainforest herbs. I did that so you would have easy access. I'm also assuming you can't go out to your garden and get these herbs. They should be available in dried form at any store that sells herbs.

Really all you need to know is to keep herbs away from metal. Use porcelain or glass. That's it. You're on your way to making an actual herbal remedy.

🌺 Yummy Relaxing Tea

Combine 1 part each: passionflower and chamomile. Add ½ part lavender and lemon balm. Throw in spearmint or peppermint (spearmint is milder) to taste and a little rose hips or orange blossom if available.

Sip and enjoy your handiwork. Notice how you are getting a delightful aroma and a great taste. As a bonus remember it's really good for you, so take it slow and enjoy!

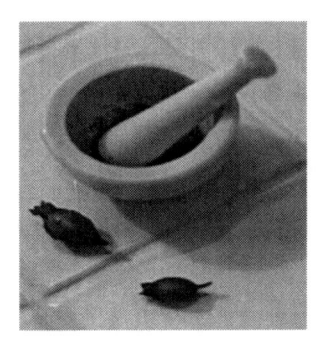

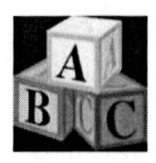

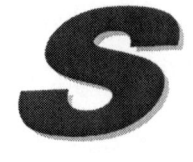

Terra Mar

S is for Sleep

*"Sleep that knits up the ravelled sleave of care
The death of each day's life, sore labour's bath
Balm of hurt minds, great nature's second course,
Chief nourisher in life's feast."* -- **William Shakespeare,** "Macbeth"

Did you know that fruit flies and ants would die if they didn't sleep? Or that our cognitive performance and mental alertness goes down with less than eight hours off the grid?

Let's consider two questions: If you have sleep issues what can you do about it? And can rainforest herbs help with your particular sleep issue?

BTW, even if you sleep well, you may find some healthful tips here.

Sleep problems. Do you qualify?

No hiding... You know who you are. Can't fall asleep, wake up during the night, can't get back to sleep. And the (groan) next day... Any of these sound familiar?

Irritable, impatient, emotional, weepy, easily bored, poor memory for simple recall, difficulty concentrating, lack of vigor, accident prone, inattentive...

No, I'm not describing your ex.

If you experience these occasionally, that makes you human. If you experience them regularly, you've got sleep issues. The National Sleep Foundation estimates direct and indirect impacts on the economy from sleep disorders and resultant daytime sleepiness at *over $100 Billion/year*. (!)

Sleepyheads cause over 100,000 traffic accidents per year.

Up to 90 percent of patients with depression have sleep issues.

Sleep deprivation affects health in other ways as well. It slows down wound healing, hits the immune system, and slows both memory and metabolism.

The good news is that most of us have the opportunity to increase the chance of a good night's sleep with some adjustments.

The following four pointers may help:

🌿 Don't overstimulate yourself

Most of us won't stimulate ourselves with caffeine late in the evening. But we will watch the news, an edge-of-the-seat thriller, or a horror film before going to bed. Not good! It's the equivalent of putting Red Bull into your system for a nightcap.

Note to self: Adrenaline doesn't care if we put a physical upper into our system or an emotional one. It can't tell the difference and produces exactly the same way.

❧ Make pre-sleep adjustments

If you have trouble falling asleep at night, reconsider what your do starting two or even three hours before bedtime. That entails reviewing all stimuli including heavy meals and alcohol. Take into consideration as well what you do right before you sleep. Is it restful, or sleep-inducing?

❧ Take power naps

Counterintuitive though it may seem, the short so-called power nap does not affect the 'circadian rhythms' that dictate our natural sleep patterns. They are actually good for us because it's a way to decrease stress and improve productivity.

❧ Listen to the master

We really do have internal clocks; that one's not just an odd idiom. Our clocks determine whether we are morning birds or night owls. They regulate blood pressure, blood temperature and metabolism. These are controlled by the little Swiss watchmaker in our brain, the Master Clock (MC).

The MC is comprised of some 20,000 neurons located near the optic nerve that together help us 'see', and adapt to the changing demands of night and day. Each day our optic nerve connects with our master clock to reset it. Once the 20,000 neurons of the MC are in agreement about our rhythms, they pass the info around the neighborhood until every one of our cells gets the latest time data. Our bodies are so amazing!

Given this sensitive, complex process it can be hard on us as we adapt to the sleep demands of jobs, changing shifts, friends, and frequent travel across time zones. Too much of overriding the MC, and we are likely to be visited by headaches, insomnia and a long list of other complaints.

Bottom line

For sleep to be the restorative health-balancing episode Nature intended, we really do well to follow our own rhythms. If you notice that after a few days off you're either up late at night or early to bed, you've come home to your very own circadian rhythm and made your master clock and all your little clocks very happy.

Believe me; I know you can't always do this. As a circadian night owl I'm all too aware of that. I think you morning birds have it easier. For years I had to wake up at 6:50 a.m. Monday through Friday. I learned to keep two alarms – one well out of the danger zone of arms' reach. I had to; there are only so many times you can tell the boss you overslept.

By Saturday I'd be well into my normal late night rhythm and sleep in on Sunday morning. I dreaded Sunday nights because I knew I would never get to sleep in time to feel like a functioning human being on Monday morning.

Anecdotal study: This shows up early and doesn't change. I don't think I mentioned that my boys are fraternal twins. They always got along wonderfully although they have different personalities. They also have different sleep patterns.

When they were little, the one who takes after me in sleep patterns would get crazed the more tired he got. His brother would be the one to put the skids on it. He'd just stand there looking forlorn and say "I'm tired. Let's go to bed now," and off they'd go. He's still the morning bird.

How much sleep do we need?

Without getting deeper into the science of it, remember that how many hours we sleep is far less important than *when* we sleep. That said, major studies indicate with less than eight hours our cognitive abilities decrease making complex reasoning and recall difficult.

Studies also show that waking naturally after seven or even six hours is also healthy. With the caveat that you are waking naturally, it seems for health purposes, the optimum number of hours is actually around seven.

If you think you've got sleep issues, consider the dolphin and take heart. We think of them as happy creatures who love to play. But either they don't get enough sleep, or they've conquered it. Dolphins allow one half of their brain to go to sleep while the other half remains awake. (Reminds me of many a Monday morning). They do this in two-hour cycles until they meet their day's sleep need. Sounds pretty Yoda-like, don't you think?

Sleep aids

When I went through cancer treatment I could have gotten any legal feel-good drug on the planet. One of the prescriptions I did get was for Ambian. Part of the reason was that with my chemo I got a steroid that kept me up, like all night. I decided to try the pill. Once was enough for me. You may be different.

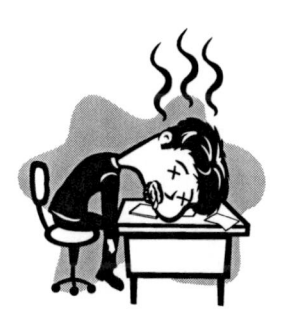

In normal sleep we go back and forth in half-hour increments between REM and non-REM sleep. In REM sleep we dream, we move, our heartbeat, breathing, and blood pressure is like when we're awake. In non-REM we're zombied out.

This doesn't happen with sleeping pills. It skips the REM, and keeps us zombied out.

I could have dealt with feeling groggy the next day. I had plenty of days when I didn't feel great. What I couldn't deal with was that for exactly six hours I was dead and then at exactly six hours and one second I woke up with a start. It felt totally unnatural. I'm not saying you would react that way. Some folks love it.

As for me, I took up a search for natural sleep aids. If you want something with a reputation for helping people relax, promoting sleep, is non-addictive and doesn't leave you feeling groggy, here are my suggestions for tried, tested and much-loved rainforest herbs. You have been introduced to these in other chapters.

Mulungu was introduced in **F is for Fatigue**. I adore mulungu and have relied on it for everything from gently taking off the edge to helping with sleep. I have heard from many users that they love it too.

Catuaba, again. I highlighted catuaba in **A is for Aphrodisiac** as well as **F is for Fatigue**. It is best known for its aphrodisiac qualities, but is a wonderful herb to help with anxiety and exhaustion. Like my young son, we sometimes get wired when we're tired and can't sleep when we need it most. This helps us rest. It's also used for forgetfulness and poor memory, common symptoms of fatigue.

Damiana is similar to catuaba in that it is appreciated both for its aphrodisiac qualities and is recommended as a support of anxiety, depression and restful sleep.

Passionflower. Such a yummy plant. It has large, magnificent flowers. It provides passion fruit, which is a delicacy. And its flowers, leaves, and stems have been used for hundreds of years for pain, to settle the nerves, and to treat insomnia. A magnificent sensory gift with sedative effects, and due to its natural serotonin, anti-depressant capabilities as well.

Yawn. Sleepy time thoughts and activities:

Ideally get a pen and paper for this. You know the definition of insanity is doing the same thing today that you did yesterday and expecting different results. If you really want to sleep better, you may have to seriously take on some habit change.

Change can be pesty, but it also spices up our lives

- What do you usually do 2 -3 hours before bed? Think back over the past few nights, and jot down notes. If you write you may be surprised at what comes out. Consider some *realistic* new wind-down habits. Perhaps drink a relaxing tea in place of soda and munchies. Read something calming. Meditate. Listen to soothing music. Take a bath.

    I don't know what works for you. *But you do.*

- What do you bring into your bedroom? Computer? Ton of books? TV? Snoring partner? Oy. *Don't.*

Terra Mar

- Give your bedroom a sleep-well Feng Shui onceover. What does the ideal sleeping room look like for you? Is it darker, quieter, painted a different color? What is in there to make it more soothing?

    Commit to making the most essential changes.

- Remember your bedroom is meant for sex and sleep.

    Keep the rest of the world at bay.

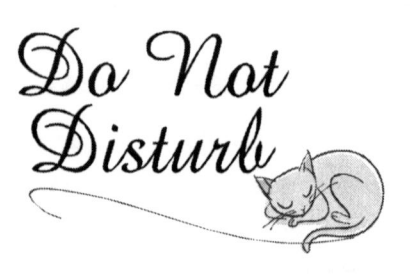

Do Not Disturb

T is for Trees

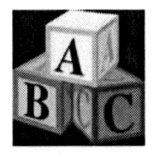

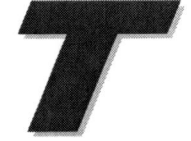

"Leaf wisdom – of change, ever releasing
Branch wisdom – of growth, ever reaching;
Root wisdom – of endurance, ever deepening."
– **Jen Delyth**, Celtic Journal

Trees cry out for metaphor – as in the 'Tree of Life' or 'Family Tree.' They remind us of the seasons of time as they go through their own cycle of life, death and re-birth. There are an astounding numbers of myths and fairy tales that include trees, reminding us of the old spirit connection between our two kingdoms. Of course there is ongoing scientific research on trees as well.

No matter which lens you're looking through, trees are remarkable inhabitants of the earth. They offer us a multitude of gifts and are deserving of our stewardship and respect. If our species is to survive, we would do well to reconsider our love affair with the chainsaw and rekindle the ancient sense of awe, respect and wonder we once felt for trees.

When I first lived in Vienna in a small apartment, there was one window where I could see green when I looked out. Nature's only salve for me amid a sea of concrete and brick. Four young trees grew close to my window and I watched them through the seasons that first year. I was so excited when the fresh leaves came again in early spring.

One morning I woke to the sound of a chainsaw outside my window. I leapt out of bed to see the beginning of the destruction of the trees. One young tree had already been cut and the workmen were on a break. With no breeze in the air and no further activity I saw the fresh spring leaves on the remaining trees shaking so strongly that I woke my husband to make sure I wasn't fantasizing their fear. We looked and wept. It was almost 30 years ago and I remember them still.

Old, older, ancient

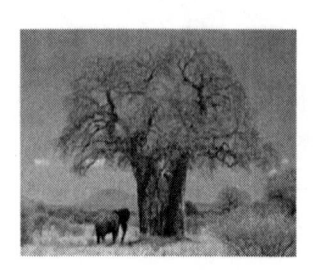

Do you know the oldest trees on earth? If you answered California Redwood you'd be close, but wrong. The oldest verifiably measured tree is the African Baobab, (*Adansonia digitata*), which carbon dating places at *6,000* years of age. The Baobab survives and thrives in one of the most hostile climates on earth, the hot, dry savannahs of sub-Saharan Africa. It is more than a metaphor for survival against the odds.

It's not especially beautiful as trees go, but consider what it offers in a climate where bare-bones survival is a challenge.

Its fruit has twice as much calcium as milk, it is high in anti-oxidants, iron and potassium, and has six times the vitamin C of an orange. Dissolved in milk or water, the fruit can be used as a drink. The leaves can be eaten as relish. The seeds produce edible oil.

In 2008, the European Union approved the use and consumption of baobab fruit as an ingredient in cereal bars and smoothies. PhytoTrade Africa, a non-profit organization, plans to market the fruit for the benefit of 2.5 million of the poorest families in southern Africa.

By ring count the Bristlecone Pine (*Pinus longaeva* – no kidding!) species includes the oldest living tree. Like the Baobab it is remarkable not only in age, but in habitat. These pines live at over 10,000 feet above sea level, in thin air and rocky earth, with incessant winds and a growing period of less than two months.

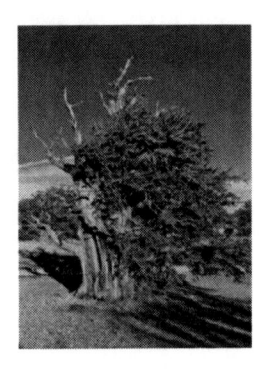

The oldest, dubbed Methuselah is now 4,848 years old. In the 1950's a researcher was trying to accurately date the species. He was horrified when he counted 4,600 rings and realized he had just killed one of the earth's oldest living beings to study it.

The exact whereabouts of Methuselah is being kept secret to protect it from a similar fate.

How about the tallest tree? That's where the majestic coastal redwood is number one, at a tad over 379 feet. A Doug Fir in Oregon is pretty close, tipping 326 feet.

The nature of trees and trees in nature

Interesting though this info may be for tree nerds like me and perhaps many of you, the truth of trees and humans is filled with mystery, magic, and volumes of lore. Why not, when you consider what trees have to offer.

Millions of years ago, trees established themselves as the most successful plant in the competition for earth and sunlight. In return, they have remained a source of protection from predators for small animals, a cornucopia of food, and a resource for dispersing pollen and seeds.

Biologically speaking, we would not exist but for trees, as that is where the prosimians evolved and later came down from the trees as our forerunners in the form of apes and monkeys with opposable thumbs.

 Nor could we continue to exist without trees. Currently there are an estimated 400 billion trees in the world, with most of that number in the tropical rainforests.

It's a fraction of what we once had on Earth, but still enough to filter carbon dioxide, carbon monoxide, sulfur dioxide and ozone from the air and exude oxygen and water for us to use.

Remember the little factoid about 20 percent of the oxygen we breathe coming from the Amazon rainforest? Absent a sufficient number of trees our planet would lose the atmosphere of 'life supporting imbalance' we need to breathe.

One large tree can produce five pounds of oxygen a day. If you have lived in a city in summer, you'll appreciate that one tree provides the cooling equivalent of ten room air conditioners. They radiate coolness in the heat of summer, and warmth at night. They reduce run-off and protect the earth from erosion.

Other important uses we have gained from trees: Sticks for hunting, wood for hiking, masks, divination, musical instruments and firewood for warmth and cooking. Trees have helped us so much that we soon began the consumer relationship with trees that haunts us still.

We have used wood for ships, shelter, furniture, bridges, and more, but forgot along the way that whilst we were growing in numbers our allies and planetary partners were being diminished and destroyed.

As we have cut, not only have we been mindlessly destroying our most loyal ally, but we have made deep and painful cuts into the spiritual and cultural relationships between trees and humans.

Terra Mar

Spirit of the woods

Trees are the only beings believed to simultaneously inhabit the three spirit realms of heaven, earth and the underworld. This has been depicted in almost every culture as a world tree. Because of their reach into all realms, they have been magnets for religious, mystical, spiritual and scientific seekers.

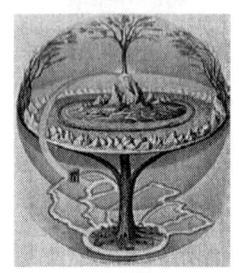

The Tree of Life was revered in ancient Egypt. The Buddha became enlightened as he meditated under a sacred fig tree. Eve ate from the apple tree while Newton understood gravity as an apple fell from the tree. Jesus was a carpenter, dependent on trees, and of course died on one.

In Judaism the Cedars of Lebanon are symbols of God's goodness. In the ascent of Muhammad, a Lote tree marked the point beyond which only Allah knew what existed and represents a manifestation of Allah.

The Yew is associated with Christianity; the Oak with Druids and Celts, the Salwa tree, representing the cosmic World Tree is sacred to Shiva. Pagans revere tree groves as holy places of worship. Native Americans tell their history on a tree, the totem.

Summer Solstice is celebrated around a decorated tree pole (the maypole). In shamanism, trees are the portal to the spirit realm.

Apologies to any group I have not represented and still I have only touched the tip of the leaf.

Trees, as I have mentioned before, are also an important source of herbs. Chuchuhuasi and jatobá are huge canopy trees. Mulungu and huanarpo macho are medium trees. Many of the amazing rainforest healers are huge vines, ferns or trees.

If we let them, trees will continue to serve us and provide for our spiritual and physical needs. They are still our allies.

They are also our collective responsibility.

Treetivities:

Do you have a tree story?

I was in Hungary at Lake Balaton several years ago for an outdoor martial arts camp where we trained several hours a day. Between our cabins and the training area were a few blocks lined with cherry trees that were filled to the brim with ripe, red cherries.

That week, amid the green leaves and red cherries the trees were lined with funny looking tree squatters dressed in white outfits. I wasn't in the habit of climbing trees after hours of training, but the trees beckoned, and we ate our way back home. They were the best cherries I ever had.

🌿 **Do you have a personal relationship with a tree?**

A favorite tree? If not, consider finding a tree and following it through the seasons. A deciduous tree is easier, but not essential. All trees show signs of the seasons.

🌿 **Keep a "Seasons Journal"**

Take note of your thoughts, inspirations, feelings, and ideas as you participate up close and personal in the amazing life cycle of a tree.

🌿 **Could you rely on a tree in tough times?**

I have.

When I went through cancer I relied on trees in many ways. A tree species that inspired me was the Alder. It is considered Nature's healer. The Alder flourishes in the most needed places -- where the earth has been damaged or polluted or where disease caused other trees to die.

As it grows, it exudes healing nitrogen into the earth. With a life span of about 40 years the Alders remain until other trees take root again, and then take a back seat.

If you need help from a tree, ask. You may be amazed if you can quiet your mind and listen. If you need a good listener some time, try telling your troubles to a tree.

U is for Upset

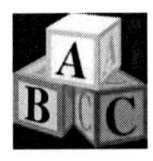

"Are you upset little friend? Have you been lying awake worrying? Well, don't worry...I'm here. The flood waters will recede, the famine will end, the sun will shine tomorrow, and I will always be here to take care of you." -- **Charlie Brown to Snoopy**

Upset can be put mapped on a bell curve. On one end are the few people who actually enjoy being upset. I don't like to spend time with them. Then there are most of us. We don't seek emotional upheaval and upset. We just accept it as a downside of being human. On the other end of the curve are the very few advanced and enlightened amongst us who have transcended upset. We pay a lot of money to be around them.

Just to make sure we're on the same page here. I'm not talking about mere digestive upset. In my case that's an artificial distinction. Ever since I was a kid, my emotional upset has headed right to my stomach. It used to be so consistent that as a young child I learned ways to figure out what had upset me. I knew once I found it, my stomach ache would go away.

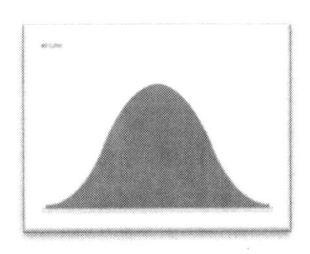

Probably not the best technique for dealing with emotional issues, but it helped me because I realized at an early age I had a direct link between my emotions and my physiology.

Am I alone in that? Not hardly! Consider for a moment, *what* is upset when we are. What happens to our physiology? Can we avoid it? What are the mistakes we make in dealing with upset?

> ❧ Those on the edge of the upset Bell curve may not even realize who they are. Here are some indicators.

Someone who:

- ✓ Walks around with a chip on their shoulder, ready for a fight

- ✓ Feels sad much of the time

- ✓ Acts grumpy and appears to have no concern for others

- ✓ Becomes overly dependent on others to make decisions and take risks because they can't do it themselves

- ✓ Constantly worries about money, health, others, or whatever is next on the list

Emotional upset & physiology

Our bodies are hardwired to deal with upset. That's the job of our endocrine system, which takes charge on a moment's notice. Our hormonal balance shifts and neurotransmitters are released. Adrenalin charges through our body; blood drops out of our digestive system and into our brain and respiratory system; endorphins are released so we don't feel pain.

We go pale, we get red, we shake, our heartbeat increases, our belly hurts, our blood pressure rises, our palms get sweaty. We are on high alert, totally prepared for flight or fight.

It's not unhealthy to get upset, even alarmed on occasion. It's not unhealthy as long as our body has the opportunity to go back to a state of relative calm.

What to do, what to do

Here are four ways that can help.

🌺 Move!

When we're in flight or fight mode we are ready to rock 'n roll. Whether flighting or fighting, we are *moving*. Beyond doubt, and as many studies have validated, movement is the most natural and healthy response to emotional and physiological upset.

I'm not endorsing fighting, by the way. Run, walk, kick or punch a non-living thing, hop up and down, shake.

Any of it helps. It not only helps the body return to a more relaxed state, it also helps deflect the potential of long-term trauma from a deeply upsetting event.

❦ Breathe!

Sometimes we don't have the privacy to move around. But we can focus on the breath. Return the breath to an even in and out rhythm. Four counts in, four counts out, till the breathing slows. Bring it down to six.

Remember: *It is not physiologically possible for the body to be in a state of upset while the breath is slow and calm.*

❦ After that...

Use any of the tools in your toolbox marked soothing:
Listen to music.
Repeat a mantra.
Take a bath.
Use self-hypnosis.
Take relaxing herbs.

Tinctures are best as they work fastest and bypass the digestive system. The oldest stand-by is the famous Bach Flower Rescue Remedy.

It may not do the whole deal if your physiology is really up there, but it will definitely help. A relaxing tea is a support, but not enough for serious upset.

Rainforest herbs for upset

Mulungu, passionflower, and **damiana** are all mentioned in **S is for Sleep**, so I won't extol their virtues again. I will simply repeat that they work, they are non-addictive, and they are safe.

No relaxing herb should be required on a day-in, day-out basis. If that's what's happening, it's probably time to take a look at options for life-style changes. That said, these are wonderful herbs, well deserving of recognition and they help soothe the central nervous system so our sympathetic nervous system can help us out of our tree.

OK, fine. We have a bunch of good ideas here for dealing with emotional upheaval and upset. But what if we don't recognize the signs? What if we do, but it just keeps coming?

Stressors in my life? Ha!

Let's say you're driving to work and some moron chatting on his cell cuts you off, almost causing an accident.

Most likely you curse him out, yell some, tell the person on the other end of your cell what happened, or the passenger with you, if you're one of the laudable carpoolers. You focus again on the road, and slowly your anger recedes.

Terra Mar

That is until you get to the office a short while later and the boss dumps on you about *her* memo she thought *you* were supposed to have done. You think of answering, but instead reflect on your credit card debt and go back to your desk. Pissed.

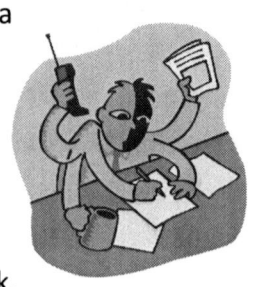

You start to feel better when the phone rings. It's the client, wondering where the memo is… Even if you've never had a day like that, you get my point, yes? We could probably follow most people through a typical day and find repeated triggers *without the ability to really calm down in between*. This may help explain why antacids are America's most popular over-the-counter remedy.

The simple fact is the flight or fight response, so incredibly powerful, and so easily tripped in humans is entirely *inappropriate* for coping with the day-to-day stresses of modern 21st century life. It's overkill; we're not beating off a tiger at the mouth of the cave anymore.

Instead we're coping with many non-life threatening stressors that nevertheless induce the same life-saving fight or flight reflex. If we don't recognize that our physiology has jumped and bring ourselves back to equilibrium, we eventually live in an ongoing stressful state. That causes nothing you or I would want.

These not-good results include, but are not limited to a weakened immune system, chronic fatigue, hypertension, poor digestion, overtaxed adrenals, and ongoing nervous upset.

That list however is incomplete. Many of society's worst scourges are actually coping mechanisms by enough individuals to cause an epidemic. This includes alcoholism and other drug addictions, obesity, anorexia and other eating disorders, violence, smoking, and insomnia.

You do not have to be part of the growing statistics. You have come all the way to **U** in your quest for a better life. Stay conscious. Check inside. Use natural means to support yourself. Let positive change happen.

Tools to help with Upset:

🌿 **Food**

Que nutrient-rich food. You probably knew it was coming, but it does keep your body healthy so it rebounds more easily. The regular applies -- fresh fruits and vegetables, especially in season; organic as much as possible, but especially if you eat meat fish, eggs, or dairy. Vitamin B is important.

Munch nuts, sunflower and other seeds for a snack instead of pastries, sweets, salty and other artificial foods.

Terra Mar

- **Recognize the signs of upset in yourself.** Remember that often people don't even know they're upset. Become more conscious of your responses.

- **Recognize the people and situations that upset you.** Recognition alone won't be enough, but there's no way to start without it.

- **Use the move and breathe techniques** as your first line of readjustment, even if it's for a few brief moments.

- **Create your own soothing toolbox.** Find what works for you. These should be enjoyable. Practice. Begin using them to cope with relatively low stress situations and use them regularly so they're available when you really need them.

- **Use relaxing herbs you trust.** Have relaxing teas around. Make sure you're really relaxed before you sleep at night. The relaxing herbs mentioned in **S is for Sleep** are great allies.

V is for Virus

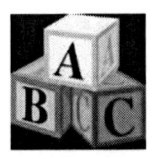

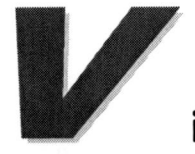

"What more fiendish proof of cosmic irresponsibility than a Nature which, having invented sex as a way to mix genes, then permits to arise, amid all its perfumed and hypnotic inducements to mate, a tireless tribe of spirochetes and viruses that torture and kill us for following orders?" – **John Updike** (1932-2009)

What's life without a cell?

If you adhere to the standard definitions of life – a being with a cellular structure that needs fuel to survive and reproduces, you may legitimately question whether or not a virus is a life form or simply an organism that interacts with life forms. It's made of simple proteins and RNA and sometimes DNA as well.

Some consider viruses to be 'organisms at the edge of life.' Whatever you label these guys, they are a force to be reckoned with. Measuring in at about 100 times smaller than bacteria, their ability to thrive and survive is off the charts. They're opportunistic, patient, and frequently die for their cause. Gee, that almost sounds human!

Terra Mar

Simple in form, their workings are complex, efficient, and generally overpowering to whatever cell they take hold of. Unable to move on its own, a virus floats around until it finds a host cell.

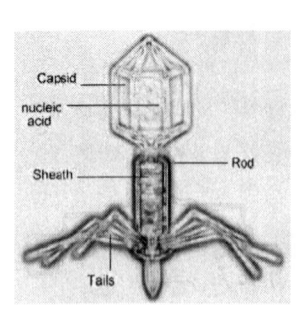

Then it docks, injects a little RNA into the cell, and in no time it's in the driver's seat. The cell continues its other functions, but adds a startling new one. It produces viruses within it. Millions of them.

The cell may die a natural death, which 50 to 70 billion of our cells do each day. Or it may valiantly commit cell suicide (a-pop-tosis) if it is aware it has been occupied.

Or the virus may order it around demanding it stay alive longer or die sooner. As the dying host's outer membrane tears open it releases out into the body the millions of viruses that have assembled inside it.

Each one goes looking for a new host cell. This is sounding like a sci fi flick, but it's happening right now.

You'd think at that rate we'd be overcome with any virus that enters our body. Of course we're not, and all in all that feels like a miracle. But remember our amazing immune system (**I is for Immune**).

Like cancer cells, viruses float around inside of us and generally are held in check. As long as they don't dock and multiply it's all good.

Most times even when a virus does take hold our immune system figures out how to build an antibody and marches us right into battle. While it's figuring it out, we feel rotten.

Typically with the most common viruses we also sneeze and cough. And guess who's in those tiny spit balls looking for another host?

The viral bucket

We can protect against some viruses, mostly with vaccinations like flu shots or the Salk vaccine against the polio virus. But we have a long way to go to cope with these guys. Our research is truly in its infancy.

It wasn't until 1955 that a woman identified the complete structure of a virus. In 1963 Hepatitis B was identified, and in 1983, HIV. So far, mostly in the latter half of the 20th century we've identified 2,000 viruses.

It's really no more than a drop in the viral bucket. There are more different types of viruses than plants, animals or bacteria.

Plenty are benign, but enough cause us multitudes of ills and evils including the common cold and flu, chickenpox, herpes, HIV/AIDS and SARS. Viruses are even being considered in MS, chronic fatigue syndrome and mental illness.

Most scientists believe viruses have been around as long as there have been cells, so as long as life itself. With such a successful species it's a safe bet they're pretty flexible, dodgy and mutable.

Viruses take this to a whole new level. They are expert players at hide-and-seek using various mechanisms to transpose themselves. The results can be devastating.

They can do the 'genetic drift,' changing their own DNA or RNA base. That's how they resist antiviral drugs.

They can also dance the 'antigenic shift,' whereby they make a major change to their own genome by assembling themselves in a new way.

In a flu virus that can lead to a pandemic. Just when we think we've got it, whammo it mutates.

In the one year between 1918 and 1919, it is estimated we lost five percent of the world's population to the Spanish Flu. About 100 million people. Sadly, unlike a typical flu, this one attacked mainly young adults.

In the HIV/AIDS pandemic, the World Health Organization estimates more than 25 million people have already died of AIDS since it was identified in 1981.

In 2007 there were an estimated 2.7 million new infections.

Diversify or be gone with you

Have you ever wondered why diversity is so important? Study the virus and I promise you will gain a new respect for the importance of diversity, not only in our own human gene pool, but in all animals and plants.

Obviously to combat viruses -- numero uno -- is a well-developed and healthy immune system. It is equally important to keep our gene pools as diverse as possible. Celebrate different races and intermixing. It keeps our children strong! Incest has always been taboo, and there are good genetic reasons for it.

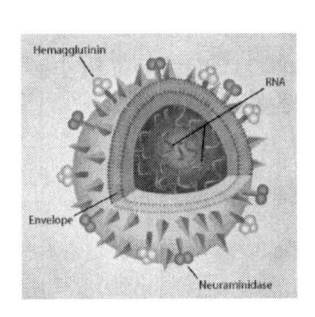

Perhaps you've noticed with pets that all purebreds are subject to the same weaknesses and illnesses. Let's pick on cats.

What if a virus came through that affected only one breed of cat? If it was severe enough we might lose that breed.

Bad enough, but *what if there were only breed of cat?* Catlovers – no worries, for now it's only an example.

In the wild animal kingdom, **diversity of food supply is** one way to ensure survival.

Consider the plight of the panda that eats only bamboo stalks. Double trouble: a limited digestive system that can only handle one food, and a reliance on only one crop. Not good.

Contrast that with the thieving raccoons in your neighborhood. As we encroach on them they eat our garbage. Now which species do you think is more likely to survive?

Hey, what about us?

Until we figure out how to survive on fresh air, lots of love and sunshine, we need a healthy food supply to help keep us healthy. The old model of a small farm with varieties of fruit, veggies, grains and animals was a highly successful sustainable model of diversity.

Studies comparing productivity on such a farm to a larger farm model have found that acre for acre the smaller, diverse farm was vastly more productive by every standard of measurement.

How can that be you may say when we genetically modify our corn or wheat, etc. to produce so much more than in the past? Ha! You've forgotten input costs and externalities. But that's a book in itself.

I simply want to point out that we're running an enormous risk to life and limb in moving to what *appears* to be a more efficient and productive approach to food supply.

If most of the corn in our Midwestern corn belt is of a few varieties, which is actually true, what in heaven's name do we do about a virus that attacks corn?

We can't risk losing all that corn (or rice or potatoes or wheat), so we spray the crop. That works for a while until the next attack. We develop a different pesticide or herbicide to fight the attacker. Runoff and pollution be damned. We need to protect our crop! Right?

Of course it's not that simple. In the monocrop world of attack – counter spray attack we are destroying the plant's ability to defend itself.

We are weakening its immune system. We are also weakening its innate intelligence and thus continuously endangering what we are trying to save. Just as a virus in a human host can bring destruction and -- writ large -- a pandemic, the same is true in the plant kingdom.

I don't know if we've forgotten or if are we so short-sighted that we're overlooking it. In either case, consider this:

One banana tree

Once upon a time there were many varieties of banana. Today we know only the sweet, soft, yellow variety. To make a long, bloody, tragic and greed-driven story short, the world is losing bananas.

The Panama Disease, for which there is no cure, is expected to kill them all within 10 to 30 years. Yes all, because they are as good as from one mother banana tree.

Maybe it's time for a rethink of how we view plants, animals and our role on this tiny planet we forget to remember is an intricate and interwoven gift.

What you can do

- For an eye-popper, read *"Banana: The Fate of the Fruit That Changed the World"* by Dan Koeppel.

- Support small farms, eat local, eat in season, grow a veggie garden. (You can even do it on your patio!)

- Rekindle your childhood connection with plants, animals and Nature by spending physical and mental time there. We protect what we feel connected to and love.

- Keep your immune system strong. Exercise, eat a good diet and get good quality cat's claw (**I is for Immune**)

- Stay away from the flu. (Good luck) If you do get one, in addition to cat's claw consider picão preto or pau d'arco. These are two tried and tested flu and cold rainforest remedies.

    Remember: your body heals you; herbs can help.

W is for Wounds

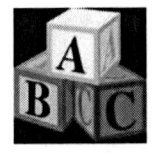

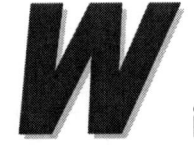

"There is something beautiful about all scars of whatever nature. A scar means the hurt is over, the wound is closed and healed, done with." -- **Harry Crews** (American writer 1935 -)

I would love to wax philosophical and chat about life's wounds and life's healings, but the **W** chapter is devoted to the body's wounds and healings. It is also dedicated to the amazing abilities of rainforest herbs to help heal those wounds.

Herbs were used to heal cuts, wounds, bites and stings of every variety long, long before antibiotics and modern medicine. Have you ever been in the tropics? Ever gotten a minor scratch that in a northern, drier climate would heal instantly? If so you know it's a wonder anything ever heals in the tropics.

My husband scratched his arm on a metal fence his second day in Costa Rica. It barely bled and he put antibiotic cream on it during his stay. Two weeks later he returned to Washington with the scratch in the very beginning stages of healing.

Within about two days if was completely healed. To this day he has a small scar.

The rainforest is an unparalleled soupy serving of bacteria, fungus and yeast. As I've mentioned, the plants that have survived and thrived there know well how to cope. Many have developed antibacterial, antifungal and antiyeast capabilities. Some have become the best at it in the world. I'd like to spotlight a few of those.

Confession: this is not only to further convince you of the inherent value of rainforest herbs. It is also because right now in the 21st century any good alternative to antibiotics is worth a try.

Off off off bacteria

Bacteria are in a tit-for-tat battle with modern science. We come up with an antibiotic. They divide, multiply and mutate. Think Broadway. Think Off Broadway, and Off Off Broadway. Now there's Off Off Off Broadway. Seriously.

That about sums up the way bacteria relate to antibiotics. As they mutate they become ever more resistant to their attacker. Since these fellows go through a generation in a few minutes, in a day they go through genetic mutations that take us humans thousands and thousands of years.

Not only are they speed demons when it comes to change. If they survive the antibiotic cure we use to kill them, they come out of the battle cheering.

That's why the doc always tells you to finish your entire course of antibiotics.

You leave one, it becomes a much stronger two, then four, eight, sixteen. In five minutes your body is greeting over a thousand of these enhanced attack agents. So it goes until you've got a vastly more resilient and tenacious bacterial infection than you started with.

Healing tips

First I'd like to offer some non-wound activities that can help you heal. The first three are real no-brainers:

- ✓ Sunlight is healing and drying, as you've surely noticed. Vitamin D helps the skin -- and much more! A caution about new scars though – keep them out of the sun for several months or they go dark.

- ✓ Exercise helps speed wound healing. This is especially true in older folks. As things slow, so does the healing process. Regular exercise improves and speeds healing by as much as 25 percent.

- ✓ Eat healthy while healing. Your body needs all the nutrients it can get, and you want the new cells to be strong.

Many complimentary techniques also support wound healing. Here are two of my favorites.

Hypnotherapy has been shown to speed healing in hand surgeries, post-birth vaginal tears, and C-sections.

Acupuncture helps boost local circulation and helps avoid scar tissue.

Show stoppers

Sangre de grado, dragon's blood (Croton lechieri). In **A is for Aphrodisiac** I introduced the "Doctrine of Signatures." This is similar. When the trunk of the dragon's blood tree is cut or wounded, a dark red, sappy resin oozes out. It's as if the tree is bleeding, and it is exactly this 'blood' that helps stop our bleeding.

Not only does it staunch bleeding, it also kills bacteria and fungi. It kills viruses, reduces pain and inflammation, and relieves itching. And it forms a thin layer, like a second skin, that seals the wound to prevent infection. According to a site monitored by a Peruvian botanist and devoted exclusively to this one herb, "Scientists have since found that as a little as a single drop of Sangre de Drago can diminish pain resulting from insect bites and stings, lacerations, burns, and plant reactions for up to six hours."
(http://www.sangrededrago.net/company.html)

These benefits have come to us through the centuries with no contraindications and no side effects. The worst that can happen? Dragon's blood could stain your clothes red. Then again, so can blood.

Scarlet bush (*Hamelia patens*) grows up to about three meters (8+ feet) in S. America and has bright reddish flowers, hence the name. It is very adaptable and is becoming popular in the southern U.S. as a landscape bush – but it only grows to about half its rainforest size. In the same family as cat's claw, it shares some of its healing properties.

Leaves are used to stop bleeding, for sores, rashes, burns, itching, cuts, skin fungus, and insect stings and bites. It also relieves pain and is anti-inflammatory. Like dragon's blood this plant has been widely used for centuries with no contraindications or side effects.

Wandering botanist Jim Conrad recounts a conversation with a Mayan healer where she recommends combining it with pomegranate and guava into a wash tea to cure skin soars as well as a mouthwash for inflammation. "And," she adds, "if you cut yourself, you heal better if you toast its leaves…, grind them to a fine powder, and sprinkle the powder in the wound." (http://www.backyardnature.net/n/08/080901.htm)

Bellaco-Caspi (*Himatanthus sucuuba*) This is another amazing rainforest herb that has been getting some recent attention in the north. In Brazil, the bark and milky white latex of this tree have been used for healing inflammations, arthritis and tumors. It is a wound healer that is antibacterial, antifungal and anti-inflammatory.

I'm only highlighting three herbs, out of several outstanding candidates. Moreover, each of these has many other functions, internally as well as externally. While research continues to provide scientific validation for traditional wisdom, the process is far from ideal.

Unfortunately if a company cannot patent some part of a plant it's not going to spend time and money to research it. It may be understandable from a business perspective, but I find it deeply regrettable for individual and planetary health.

Final wound note

Especially if you are dealing with surgical wounds or very deep wounds, give yourself time to heal. Our bodies begin the astoundingly complex process of healing from the moment a wound occurs. Sometimes this calls for a level of patience we don't ordinarily need.

Like Nature itself, healing has no straight lines. There's a lot going on inside that you may not even notice.

Stay positive and avoid stress. Relax. Rest. Check in, but also give in! Even if you feel good, don't push too hard.

Our body is designed to seek health, balance and self-healing. Let it.

Wounderful activities:

🌿 Have you ever had surgery or a bad wound? What worked? How long did it take? Did you do anything to help or hinder the process?

🌿 Looking back, is there anything you might have done different?

🌿 Look again at the healing tips. Next time you have a wound, add at least two of these to your healing process.

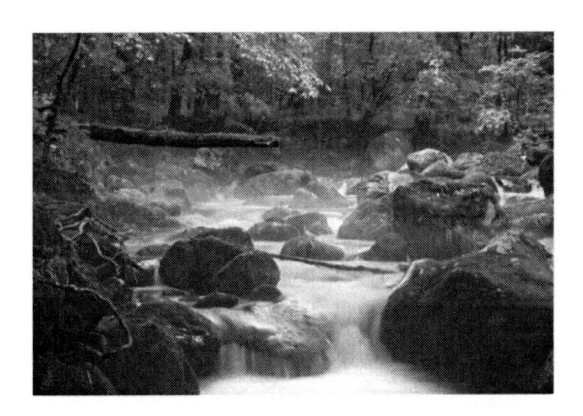

Terra Mar

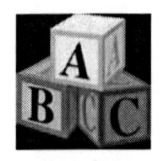

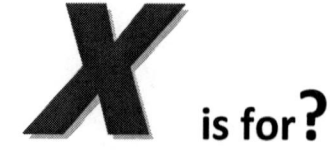

X is for ?

"Did St. Francis preach to the birds? Whatever for? If he really liked birds he would have done better to preach to the cats." -- **Rebecca West,** English writer (1892 – 1983)

? is the **X-factor**. It's the Great Unknown; the part I can't know or intuit. Neither can anyone else – except you. I can write about planetary health, natural healing, and rainforest herbs till the cows come home. I might be pleased -- more likely exhausted -- but what else happens? That's where you come in, my X-factor friend.

This ABC book was designed to offer tips, activities and ideas to help stimulate your imagination and suggest activities you might find of interest.

I'd like to take **X** to help ensure that when you walk away from this book you also take a new view of yourself. After all, we're very close to **Z**, and our time together is drawing to a close.

This is not an exam and I'm not expecting to see the results – although that would be fun. This is your letter, and my goals are simple:

ABC's of Natural Healing

Help you find, remember, deepen or renew what spoke to you and why it was important to you.

Provide a forum for you to create an activity that might bring rainforest herbs or planetary healing right to your doorstep.

X = You. It's a blank until you make of this letter what you will.

Please feel free to draw, scribble, write with your non-dominant hand... whatever allows you to really chew on this and make it your own. Remember – This is not a test and no one is watching!

My favorite letter was: _____

I liked/loved it because:_____
_____
(it changed my perspective, I got new info, I smiled)

The thought of this idea really upset me:_____
_____

And here's what I intend to do about it: _____
_____

Terra Mar

What I'm going to most remember from this book is:_____
_____

My favorite activity was:_____
_____

because I:_____
_____

In flipping back through the alphabet just now, this caught my attention: _____
_____

because: _____
_____

If I were to own one rainforest healing herb it would be: _____

If I were to change one attitude or undertake one activity to improve my health it would be: _____
_____

If I were to change one attitude or undertake one activity to help the planet more than I do right now, it would be: _____

_____

I've already begun doing this for my health: _____
_____

Color the star for that! ☆

I've already begun doing this for the Earth: _____
_____

A star to you for that as well! ☆

I am deeply grateful that : _____
_____

Now it's freestyle. Take time for additional reflection, ideas, rants, raves, dreams…… It's nothing now. Go ahead and make something of it.

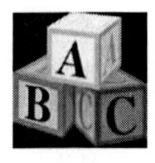

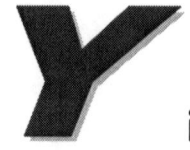

Terra Mar

Y is for Yeast

"I am personally convinced that one person can be a change catalyst, a 'transformer' in any situation, any organization. Such an individual is yeast that can leaven an entire loaf." -- **Stephen R. Covey** (Author, "Seven Habits of Highly Successful People," which has sold over 15 million copies in 20 years.)

Yeast ranges from the friendly and as in baking, beer, wine or kombucha fermentation; to functional as in biotech and alternative electricity; to the pathogenic as in Candidiasis and other yeast infections.

Of course yeast get off on sugar as anyone knows who has watched it thrive while baking bread. Then it proceeds to strongly modify the substance, which is fine if it's bread or beer. It's not at all fine if it's the normally healthy ecobalance in your intestines, lungs or vagina.

Confession: I'm writing this after ingesting a chocolate chip cookie. My diet would be so much healthier without sugar and chocolate, but, sigh, I'm still a work-in-progress. I probably just gave the Candida albicans of my world a movable feast. Bummer.

Anyway, let's talk about Candida, yeast infections, how to avoid them, and how to heal if you have one.

Note to guys: If you think because you don't get vaginal infections you're off the Candida hook, uh uh. Yeast is egalitarian and lives in the intestines and elsewhere in the bodies of women and men alike. If you've heard of 'thrush,' that is none other than a Candida infection in the mouth. General indicators and health tips apply equally to both sexes.

What yeast wants and what you don't want to give it

Three major areas support yeast infections.

✓ **Antibiotics**

Yeast loves it when you take antibiotics, especially if you don't hurry and rebuild your intestinal flora ASAP. Yeast infections are on the rise, which adds strength to the **V is for Virus** and **W is for Wounds** point of avoiding antibiotics when possible.

The healthy bacteria in our intestinal flora tend to hold the yeast at bay. Absent that, our healthy acidic balance turns overly-alkaline and makes yeast comfy.

Most antibiotics wipe out the protective bacteria that normally inhabit the vagina. Broad spectrum antibiotics are the best at it. Statistics vary, but minimally 25 percent of women will get a yeast infection after taking a course of antibiotics and it could be as high as 70 percent.

✓ Sugar

There is no doubt that a sugar-rich diet can lead to yeast infections. That includes eating a lot of the simple carbs found in white flour and junk food. One theory on junk-food and sugar cravings is that we are driven by our own Candida.

The theory posits that many of us have Candida overgrowth without being aware of it. Because of that, we maintain the same poor eating habits that tipped us into the imbalance originally.

We find ourselves in a vicious cycle, unable to change our eating habits because we are used to obeying our Candida-based cravings. This could be one of the many reasons diets are so pathetically unsuccessful over the long-term.

✓ Compromised immune system

 Of course we can't always have our immune system in top form. Any serious illness will compromise it. If we are coming off a bad flu or any of the other ills that may find us, it is important to make a conscious effort to beef up our immune system. We certainly want to keep it as strong as possible as long as possible.

Etcetera

Those are the main ones. Others include slow metabolism, not enough stomach acid, overly alkaline intestinal tract, stress, and ongoing fatigue. These factors can be mitigated by the basics, the ABC's of healthy living – a good nutrient-rich diet, good sleep and regular exercise. Aside from cravings and yeast infections, Candida overgrowth can show up as a host of seemingly unrelated symptoms in many different parts of the body or as mood swings, fatigue, weight gain and headaches.

Guys can skip this section

(Yeah, right). Women, you probably already know this stuff, but it's worth mentioning. Yeast thrives in warm damp places, so here are a few tips for keeping the balance in your favor and helping to avoid vaginal yeast infections: Breathable underwear – boring cotton undies are best; minimally panties should have a cotton crotch.

Nighttime is a good time to get fresh air on your genital area. Yeast hates that. A nightgown or longer Tee is better than jammie bottoms. After swimming or a bath, make sure you dry thoroughly. Also, keeping the intestinal flora healthy helps improve the vaginal environment as well.

What to do?

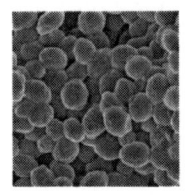

In the yeastivities below I've given a simple overgrowth test that some naturopaths use. If you think you have Candidiasis, don't panic. Some estimates are that up to 90 percent of adults have Candida overgrowth. Consult your naturopath or other health care provider. If you have Candidiasis in addition to whatever else you choose, you will have to face your food demons. Otherwise it will return.

There are many tips for anti-Candida diets, but you know the basics – out with the sugar and carbs, in with the nutrient-rich foods. The real issue is not that we don't know; it's whether we've had enough pain and suffering to shore up the political will to make change happen.

One rainforest herb in particular is a powerful Candida killer. Perhaps you've heard of it:

Pau d'arco (*Tabebuia impetiginosa)* is among the best known, most researched and most widely used of all Amazon rainforest herbs. It has been used for thousands of years. Today, in addition to combating Candida, it is commonly prescribed for skin problems, allergies, flu, upper respiratory infections, even the common cold, and more.

There are some areas of agreement about what pau d'arco has and how it works. The University of Maryland Medical Center, which publishes articles about herbs using amazing numbers of qualifications says:

"Pau d'arco contains chemical compounds called naphthoquinones such as lapachol that may have antifungal, antiviral, and antibacterial properties, as well as significant amounts of the antioxidant quercetin."

As to Candida, pau d'arco's widely agreed-upon strength as an immune builder can sock the yeast with a double whammy. By helping to kill it off, as studies seem to show, and by helping to build up the immune system, it is both curative and protective.

To give a small example of how effective pau d'arco can be, H. pylori (Helicobacter pylori) is the most common cause of stomach ulcers. Scientists were astounded to find it surviving indefinitely in the highly acidic environment of our stomachs. Western medicine treats H. pylori with a *month-long* course of antibiotics.

I know; I had it – but that was long before I discovered pau d'arco. Pau d'arco has tested positive for killing H. pylori! It has also tested successfully against several other bacteria and fungi. This includes Staph and Strep.

Know what you're using

As always, first check with your doctor. Then make sure you are getting the best quality pau d'arco you can find. Even the time of year it is harvested can affect its strength.

Also, even though many places sell it as a tea, I would recommend it as a tincture. It's the inner bark and root that is used, and generally a tea is not enough to bring out those healing qualities. They tend to be tougher than other plant parts and typically need to be boiled 10 – 20 minutes.

Jatobá has also tested well as an anti-Candida agent.

An important reminder

As with every other chapter and herb mentioned in this book, this information is purely educational. Nothing I have written is meant to replace the advice, diagnosis, care and treatment of a health care professional.

I want to underscore the point with Candida because the amount of overgrowth varies enormously among us. If you even suspect you have serious Candida problems I urge you to take the proper steps to seek out dietary and medical care.

Yeastivities:

- Take an easy test. First thing in the morning before you do anything else with your mouth – that's essential – fill a glass with water, work up some saliva and spit into the glass. Take note of how it looks after a minute or three. Then watch what happens at 15 – 30 minute intervals.

    If the saliva stays pretty much the way it was, your Candida is probably not happy.

- On the other hand, if strands form and start moving down toward the bottom, if little flecks form in the water or if saliva settles to the bottom you've probably got a lot of happy, thriving Candida and may want to look further.

- Bring a pen and paper with you the next time you go to a natural products or health food store. Write down the brand name and ingredients in the pau d'arco products. Then really take it on.

  Google the company. Call them. Write to them. Find out all you can about how they harvest, produce, and market their product.

- Be a squeaky wheel if they do not measure up to your standards. If you're still not satisfied, talk with the buyer or manager the next time you go to the store and tell them what you found out.

- If we want to hold others accountable for their products, it makes sense for us to be responsive and well-informed.

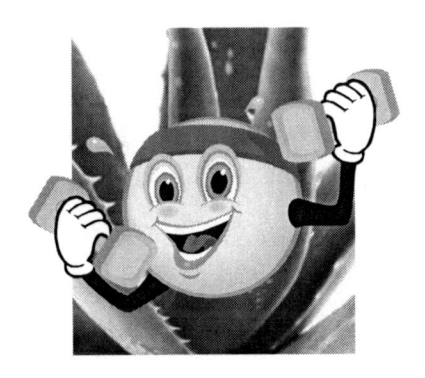

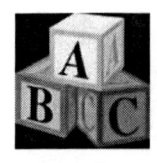

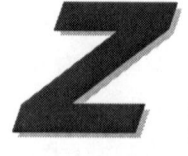

Terra Mar

Z is for Zen

"One day while walking across a field a man encountered a vicious tiger. He fled, the tiger after him. Coming to a precipice, he caught hold of the root of a wild vine and swung himself down over the edge. The tiger sniffed at him from above. Trembling, the man looked down to where, far below, another tiger was waiting to eat him. Only the vine sustained him.

Two mice, one white and one black, little by little started to gnaw away the vine. The man saw a luscious strawberry near him. Grasping the vine with one hand, he picked the strawberry with the other. How sweet it tasted." -- **Paul Reps** (1895-1990) Retelling a Japanese parable in "Zen Flesh, Zen Bones"

To Zen or not to Zen, that's not really the question. Rather in our fast-paced crazy, stressed-out, demanding world, the question is when to Zen.

If you can remain in an enlightened state of non-attachment and inner calm 24/7 not only am I totally impressed, but you're probably not reading this book. I'm thinking of the rest of us.

How do we combine the loftiest life-style concepts with constantly being thrown off our pins?

This almost feels like I'm leading up to a summary of A – Y, and in some ways, guilty as charged. Some answers are pretty obvious.

Keep moving to the center, no matter what

Most important is consistency. I expect our lives to be an active push and pull; a non-stop tug of war between tension and relaxation, joy and sadness, stuff we must do and stuff we want to do, and a whole bunch more opposites.

So how to find the still center when not in a yoga position? How to love your neighboring car when you're stuck in traffic and late for work? How to stay calm when the kids are on the ceiling?

I actually have an answer. My answer is you probably won't and that's okay as long as you come back to the still center, back to the love, back to the calm.

Sometimes we all leave our best selves stranded, thumb out hoping for a ride. It's okay not to pick up our internal hitchhiker sometimes. What matters is that we allow the wandering self to return.

It's not the leaving that requires our focus. It's the homecoming that needs our attention. Over and over.

Terra Mar

These make it easier:

Rest
Good diet
Fresh air
Contact with Nature
Cutting out stress where possible
Using relaxation techniques
Natural healing supports including rainforest herbs
Gratitude
Staying in the moment

But by **Z** you know all that and hopefully a bit more.

If you skipped **X**, hmm, please don't tell me you skipped it. If you did **X**, please revisit it. Within your sentences, or maybe hidden in the fine print and hovering between the lines are all the answers you need. **X will tell you how to heal and stay healthy.** It is your anchor to keep you safe at harbor while the storms of life rage and winds of change roar.

Zen in the art of financial crisis

As I write this, the U.S. and much of the world are locked in a downward financial spiral. The news is awful. As the American dream swirls around a new American nightmare, a lingering angst assails our positive spirits.

Worry, dread and fear are finding their way into the American Way of Life. Like much of the world I have been transfixed as the U.S. has swung into a new era with the election and inauguration of President Barack Obama.

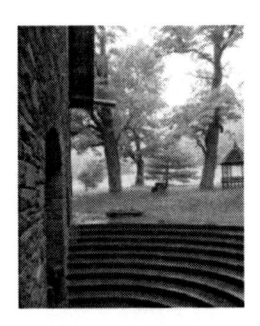

I've watched more CNN this election cycle than in my entire life combined. This despite the fact that I am too often frustrated by the superficial sound bite coverage.

But recently on CNN I heard a surprisingly in-depth discussion on many of the hard and long-term challenges facing Americans as a nation in crisis.

They talked of stopping the blame game despite our outrage. One panelist wondered whether our entitled generations will be willing to sacrifice for our children as older generations had done. Another suggested we stop throwing around the term consumer, adding we are citizens. Citizens first.

I say stewards, stewards first

It was as if the conscience – and consciousness – of a nation were finally waking from decades of sleep, struggling to be heard amidst the chaos and hysteria. A plea for conscious living in prime time? It was astounding, frightening, and exhilarating.

The talking heads were asking us to look into our collective soul and redefine what it means to be alive at this moment in history.

We have indeed turned ourselves into a nation that honors spending and deifies consumerism. Now we are being asked to change as individuals and as a society, and to change now.

It really is the perfect last letter because the implication is that is if we are going to heal, we must change. It is as true with physical healing of our bodies as with healing the Earth and biosphere that maintains us, as it is with national souls.

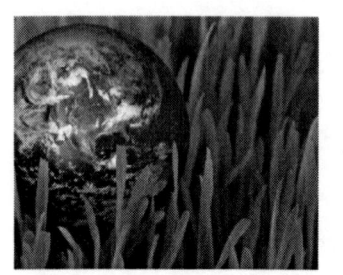

In so many ways, right now we are being asked to reconsider how we tread on this Earth and how to do better.

So many questions are crying out for answers. They range from what to do about religious conflicts, food and natural resource shortages to how to green science and technology.

Can we listen to the rhythms of the Earth and learn to dance?

The answers may not come, but as stewards, as citizens of Earth, we must keep coming back to the questions. They say every crisis is an opportunity. I would add that the larger the crisis the greater the potential opportunity.

With the power of a global crisis at our backs we can toss out what is divisive and destructive and replace it with life positives. As we move into this new era of greater consciousness and responsibility, we can heal ourselves and heal the planet.

I think it's even a little easier than that. I believe as we heal ourselves we cannot do other than to heal the planet.

Instead of a zactivity, I'll leave you with a Zen thought from one of the most profound thinkers of all time:

"A human being is part of the whole called by us Universe, a part limited in time and space. We experience ourselves, our thoughts and feelings as something separate from the rest. A kind of optical delusion of consciousness. This delusion is a kind of prison for us, restricting us to our personal desires and to affection for a few persons nearest to us.

Our task must be to free ourselves from the prison by widening our circle of compassion to embrace all living creatures and the whole of nature in its beauty... We shall require a substantially new manner of thinking if mankind is to survive."
-- **Albert Einstein**

Terra Mar

TERRA MAR has spent decades studying and working with plants. She has a unique understanding of the relationship between our health and our role as stewards of Earth.

Nature, and the in-depth study of natural healing and how plants help sustain us are her passions.

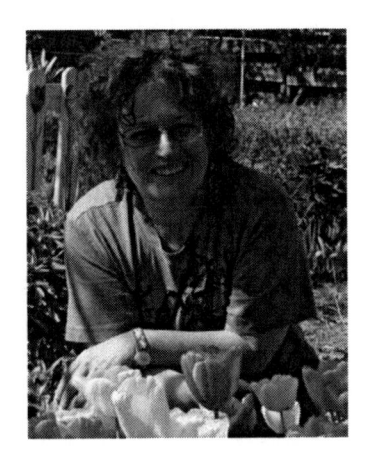

She has helped many people to lead a more balanced life, and recently expanded her activities by creating OnePlanet Herbs, where she joyfully creates Amazon rainforest remedies.

Terra freely admits to chatting with plants while making her herbal concoctions, and has travelled and written extensively on the importance of preserving and sustaining a healthy life here on planet Earth.

She can be reached at www.OnePlanetHerbs.com or at her informational site www.herbalremedies-info.com.

Please feel free to visit Terra at her websites and ask any questions of concern to you.